EMPLOYMENT LAW AND OCCUPATIONAL HEALTH

A Practical Handbo

Joan Lewis
MCIPD, Dip Law, MA (Law & Employment Relations)

Greta Thornbory
MSc, RGN, ROH, PGCEA, MIOSH

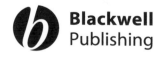

Blackwell
Publishing

Blackwell Publishing editorial offices:
Blackwell Publishing Ltd, 9600 Garsington Road, Oxford OX4 2DQ, UK
    Tel: +44 (0)1865 776868
Blackwell Publishing Inc., 350 Main Street, Malden, MA 02148-5020, USA
    Tel: +1 781 388 8250
Blackwell Publishing Asia Pty Ltd, 550 Swanston Street, Carlton, Victoria 3053, Australia
    Tel: +61 (0)3 8359 1011

First published 2006 by Blackwell Publishing Ltd

2   2006

ISBN-13: 978-1-4051-4972-3
ISBN-10: 1-4051-4972-8

Library of Congress Cataloging-in-Publication Data
Lewis, Joan, MCIPD.
Employment law and occupational health : a practical handbook/Joan Lewis, Greta Thornbory.
    p. cm.
Includes bibliographical references and index.
ISBN-13: 978-1-4051-4972-3 (pbk. : alk. paper)
ISBN-10: 1-4051-4972-8 (pbk. : alk. paper)
1. Industrial hygiene–Law and legislation–England.   2. Industrial safety–Law and legislation–England.   3. Labor laws and legislation–England.   I. Thornbory, Greta.   II. Title.

KD3168.L49 2006
344.4204'65–dc22
2006002368

A catalogue record for this title is available from the British Library

Set in 10/12.5pt Palatino
by Graphicraft Limited, Hong Kong
Printed and bound in India
by Replika Press Pvt Ltd, Kundli

The publisher's policy is to use permanent paper from mills that operate a sustainable forestry policy, and which has been manufactured from pulp processed using acid-free and elementary chlorine-free practices. Furthermore, the publisher ensures that the text paper and cover board used have met acceptable environmental accreditation standards.

For further information on Blackwell Publishing, visit our website:
www.blackwellpublishing.com

To David for happy days
and
Sam, Linda, Bernie, Mary

Joan

To Carla and the future

Greta

Contents

Foreword

Employment law relating to occupational health has evolved a long way from outlawing the sending of little boys up chimneys. The constitution of the occupational health provider has moved on from being a factory doctor assisted by a nurse to being a team of health professionals with a wide range of experience and expertise. Knowledge and understanding of employment law is now an essential component of occupational health provision.

Occupational health deals with the effects of work on health and the effects of health on the capacity to work. Work and the workplace have to be considered first as a cause or contributor to disease and second as a place to return to after illness or injury. However, as the workplace has become less dangerous and the prevalence of occupational disease has decreased, the occupational health team has become increasingly involved with the effects that health may have on work.

The employer has statutory responsibilities for the protection of the health of the workforce, as well as a general duty of care for the health and safety of employees, which extends to the highest levels of management. The increasing complexity of employment law and good work practice, together with the rising expectations of employees and their lawyers, have required managers to consult an increasingly wide range of publications and statutes to ensure the discharge of duty of care.

This new handbook is written by a highly experienced occupational health practitioner and a well respected and experienced employment law consultant. It brings together in one book a practical and pragmatic guide on employment law relating to occupational health, and will be the answer to the prayers of many managers and their colleagues. It is a book to be consulted rather than read from cover to cover, and consult it you will.

Michael Bagshaw *MB MRCS FFOM DAvMed*
Professor of Aviation Medicine, King's College London
Formerly Head of Occupational & Aviation Medicine, British Airways plc

Preface

Legal editing of this book has been provided by the following barristers:

Linda Goldman, BDS, LLB
Laura Robinson BSc (Hons), PgDL, BVC

at the Chambers of John Fitzgerald, 7 New Square, Lincoln's Inn, London. We are indebted to them for their expertise, wit and wisdom.

This book provides general guidance only and must not be regarded as providing formal legal advice or opinion.

We have included the current legal framework up to the end of 2005, with proposed and relevant legislative changes expected during 2006, in our guidance and references. We suggest that, given the pace of change in the development of employment law, the current position should always be checked. To that end we have provided website sources to assist in this aspect of ongoing professional development.

Throughout the book where the terms 'he', 'his' and 'him' are used, these should be taken to refer to both genders.

Acknowledgements

We are both indebted to so many people for their help, encouragement and support. It is not possible to name each one individually but we take this opportunity to express our gratitude to everyone who has helped us.

There are some whose names should be mentioned in acknowledgement of their contribution to our work and research: Professor Michael Bagshaw; Walter Brennan, Oliver Brennan Training Consultancy; Robert Dunn, University of Oxford Occupational Health Service; Anne Harriss; Jo Jenkins; Kay McAnulty, Capita Health Solutions; Chris Packham, Enviroderm; Neil Ridsdale and Ken Barltrop, Complywise; Suzanne Smith, Manage Absence Ltd; Dr Stuart Whitaker; Elizabeth Wilson; Melanie Wyatt, Well Aware Occupational Health Service; the Association of Occupational Health Nurse Practitioners (UK). There are others who have given their help and wish to remain anonymous.

We are grateful to Claire White for her invaluable help in the technical and editing work she has undertaken for us.

We would like to thank Beth Knight, Katharine Taylor and Richard Miles of Blackwell Publishing. Their guidance, encouragement and professional support throughout this project have been invaluable.

When we embarked upon this project together we planned our time carefully. We omitted to consider that life decides to go its own way despite those best laid plans. We have each experienced sad and happy events during the course of our work, but throughout the project we have retained our commitment, good humour and enjoyment in working together.

So, in closing, we would both like to thank all of our friends, colleagues and families. We hope they will welcome us back and forgive us for our absence while we worked on this book.

Joan Lewis
Greta Thornbory

Abbreviations

ACAS	Advisory, Conciliation and Arbitration Service
AFOM	Associate Member of the Faculty of Occupational Medicine of the Royal College of Physicians
ANO	Air Navigation Order
CAA	Civil Aviation Authority
CIPD	Chartered Institute of Personnel and Development
COSHH	Control of Substances Hazardous to Health (Regulations and Approved Code of Practice) 2002
CAB	Citizens Advice Bureau
DDA	Disability Discrimination Act 1995
DH	Department of Health
DPA	Data Protection Act 1998
DRC	Disability Rights Commission
DSS	Department of Social Security
DWP	Department for Work and Pensions
EAT	Employment appeal tribunal
EC	European Community
EMA	Employment medical advisor
EMAS	Employment Medical Advisory Service
EOC	Equal Opportunities Commission
EPA	Equal Pay Act 1970
EPCA	Employment Protection (Consolidation) Act 1978
ERA	Employment Rights Act 1996
ET	Employment tribunal
EU	European Union
GMC	General Medical Council
GP	General practitioner
HASWA	Health and Safety at Work etc. Act 1974
HAVS	Hand–arm vibration syndrome
HSC	Health and Safety Commission
HSE	Health and Safety Executive
ME	Myalgic encephalomyelitis (chronic fatigue syndrome)
MFOM	Member of the Faculty of Occupational Medicine of the Royal College of Physicians
MHSWR	Management of Health and Safety at Work Regulations
MS	Multiple sclerosis
MSP	Maternity suspension pay
NHS	National Health Service

NMC	Nursing and Midwifery Council
OH	Occupational health
OSP	Occupational sick pay
PPE	Personal protective equipment
PUWER	Provision and Use of Work Equipment Regulations 1992
RCN	Royal College of Nursing
RIDDOR	Reporting of Injury, Diseases and Dangerous Occurrences Regulations 1995
RRA	Race Relations Act
RSI	Repetitive strain injury
SDA	Sex Discrimination Act
SMEs	Small and medium-sized enterprises
SSP	Statutory sick pay
VWF	Vibration white finger
WRULD	Work-related upper limb disorder

Table of Cases

Table of Statutes

Other statutes of interest

Industrial Relations Act 1971
Occupiers' Liability Act 1957

Table of Statutory Instruments

Other legal references

Other statutory instruments of interest

Children (Protection at Work) Regulations 1998 and 2000 SI Nos. 276, 1333

Health and Safety at Work Act (Application outside Great Britain) Order 1995 SI No. 263
Health and Safety at Work (Northern Ireland) Order 1978 SI No. 1039
Health and Safety (Consultation with Employees) Regulations 1996 SI No. 1513
Health and Safety (Enforcing Authority) Regulations 1998 SI No. 494
Health & Safety (First Aid) Regulations 1981 SI No. 917
Health and Safety (Information for Employees) Regulations 1989 SI No. 682
Health and Safety (Training for Employment) Regulations 1990 SI No. 1380
Health and Safety (Young Persons) Regulations 1997 SI No. 135

Management of Health and Safety at Work and Fire Precautions (Workplace)
    Amendment Regulations 2003 SI No. 2776

Race Relations Act 1976 (Amendment) Regulations 2003 SI No. 1626
Railways (Safety Critical Work) Regulations 1994 SI No. 299

Sex Discrimination (Gender Reassignment) Regulations 1999 SI No. 1102

Introduction

Employment law and the health of employees is everyone's business. Whereas lawyers have no need to learn the skills of health professionals, in today's world everyone who advises, treats or manages people at work needs to know the basic practical aspects of employment rights.

Taking care of our health is vital to every individual and to all employers. At work the first priorities are safeguarding good health and managing absence due to illness or injury. The cost of sickness absence presents a major cost and business management problem to employers. Failure to get to grips with absence management can risk the financial health of the business and the job security of employees. The risk of expensive litigation in the courts or employment tribunals is too costly and common to be ignored by any employer today.

From our very first discussions about this book, our objectives in its writing and research were clear. We wanted to write a practical handbook on employment law relating to occupational health: a book that would be a real resource for those with any responsibility for health in the workplace and especially those advising on occupational health. With our respective backgrounds in employment law and occupational health, we have tried to bring together a uniquely common-sense guide to advising and managing workplace health.

Our handbook is intended to be a guide to the everyday issues that occur with regard to occupational health in the workplace. While it will be relevant to occupational health practitioners, it will also be a useful practical reference for general managers and human resource specialists. Where there is access to an occupational health service in the workplace, we hope the handbook will assist in a better understanding of roles, responsibilities and options in what are often very sensitive and complex situations. Where there is no occupational health service available in the workplace, we hope employers and managers who have to handle these situations without expert guidance will gain a clearer understanding of the many legal pitfalls to be avoided through following good practice with regard to employees' health problems.

We have not set out to write a legal or clinical textbook. Aside from there being many such excellent publications available, we have also been concerned to ensure that we made this handbook as useful as possible, for as long as is practically possible. The law and occupational health practice are changing and developing at a fast pace, and employment law is particularly dynamic and complex. Keeping to the aim of writing an essential resource handbook, we have tried to ensure that this guide focuses on the practical application of the key aspects of the law rather than simply the statutes and regulations. By so doing, we hope that the handbook's use will endure for a little longer than might be expected of a legal textbook.

While we have done our utmost to base our information on the latest legislative developments at the time of going to print, this handbook provides general guidance only and must not be regarded as providing formal legal advice or a comprehensive statement of the law. Each case will turn on its own facts, its individual circumstances and the law applicable at the time. We strongly suggest that whenever the need arises legal advice be obtained from an employment law specialist.

Given that our key objective was for the book to be a practical guide, we considered the fact that, so often, questions asked by occupational health professionals are to do with how they can go about their practice in order to satisfy both the employer and the employee. This may even be after conflict has arisen. In the introduction to its *Guide on Confidentiality*, the Royal College of Nursing says:

> 'To ensure the effective use of occupational health services that contribute to a healthy workforce, occupational health practitioners need to work collaboratively with both employers and workers. A clear and shared understanding of the legal and professional obligations of both practitioners and employers together with the sensitive handling of confidential information are keys to achieving this.'[1]

Today there is a minefield of legislation to step cautiously through when making decisions and giving professional advice. Occupational health practitioners have to work not only within the legislation but also within their relevant professional Codes of Practice, and at times these may seem to conflict. Often non-clinical colleagues are unaware of professional conduct issues and so may feel that occupational heath is, at best, sitting on the fence. Good practice starts with good communication and we have tried to address how clearer understanding on roles and obligations can be established from the beginning. Through a summary of legal perspectives, supported by example case studies, checklists, vignettes, sample letters and procedural guides, this book will provide readers with practical guidance on how to proceed. It will take a logical approach, considering the appropriate degree of occupational health involvement at each stage of the employment process, identifying the myths and realities of the legal requirements of employing people, providing evidence-based suggestions and giving examples of good practice.

One of the first priorities of any occupational health practitioner must be to know about company policies – what they are, where they are available and how they relate to occupational health. Secondly, it is important for the occupational health service to make efforts to be involved in developing and reviewing policies that have implications for the service. In this computerised age many companies make all personnel policies available on line via the company intranet, and so reference can be made to them at anytime. However, the reality still is that many occupational health practitioners are not aware of company policy and have not challenged, contributed to or otherwise influenced personnel practice. Is it therefore any wonder that conflict and uncertainty arise from time to time?

We have written this handbook to follow the logical steps of the employment cycle and to deal with many of the issues that may occur. Starting from pre-employment, we move through record keeping and reports, to health surveillance, occupational health services, absence and rehabilitation, and finally on to termination of employment.

Each chapter outlines some key employment rights and provides case law examples to assist and guide on those rights in practice. Key employment issues are considered, such as discrimination, data protection, working abroad, pregnancy and maternity leave, workplace policies, drugs and alcohol testing, stress, counselling, health surveillance and professional conduct rules.

We hope that this is a book readers will enjoy and find useful. We have certainly endeavoured not to write in 'legalese' or clinical jargon. We hope the book finds a place in your office and rarely sits on the shelf for long. Above all, we hope it will help towards best practice at work, business success and respect for individual employment rights.

Reference

1. Royal College of Nursing (2004) *Confidentiality: RCN Guidance for Occupational Health Nurses.* RCN, London.

Chapter 1

Recruitment and Pre-employment Health Assessment

Employing people is a function that can involve any number of persons responsible for all or part of the decision making process. In some organisations this responsibility can be vested in just one appointing person who will be the successful candidate's direct manager, while in other situations there may be a multidisciplinary team of people involved including, for example, human resources and/or external recruitment agencies, working with an occupational health service provision. Occupational health may be asked to provide an assessment of the applicant's suitability, in terms of their health, for the post for which they have applied, based on the information provided by the candidate and prospective employer. There is much more that needs to be considered, particularly from the legal perspective, not only to comply with existing legislation but also to avoid future problems both for the employer and for the health of the worker. This chapter will address the key legal issues of recruitment and pre-employment, highlighting the important role management and occupational services can play in preventing potential problems and promoting a healthy workforce.

Employment law perspectives

The recruitment process begins to have legal implications from its very outset. Following good practice in a pre-considered and standard format each time appointments are planned can avoid many pitfalls and potential legal costs that might otherwise arise.

All too often problems occur when the employing organisation considers that the legal aspects of recruitment only become relevant when an offer of employment is to be made. In fact the wording of the job advertisement, any job description details provided, the title of the job, the person specification skills and experience quoted, all have legal implications that need to be considered by employers long before offers of employment or contracts are issued.

Once the employee joins the organisation, the recruitment process is still not quite completed: the written contract of employment must be issued together with key policy documents, such as the health and safety policy, staff handbook, internal discipline, grievance and appeals procedures, equal opportunities and anti-discrimination policies, etc. Today these policies can often be found on the company intranet and so are readily available to most workers. Training and induction are vital requirements to be carried out as soon as possible so as to complete the recruitment process.

Fire and emergency procedures training are very important requirements in induction training, along with other training on policies and procedures, use of equipment generally and any particular risks and hazards.

Employees have to be trained in 'fire precautions', which are the subject of legal requirements under specific fire precautions legislation. These include the Fire Regulations and the Fire Precautions Act 1971 and, more generally, health and safety legislation including the Health and Safety at Work etc. Act 1974 (HASWA) and its subordinate regulations, as well as more specific health and safety legislation such as the Dangerous Substances and Explosive Atmospheres Regulations 2002 (DSEAR).

The Fire Regulations and the Fire Precautions Act 1971 (and Northern Ireland equivalents) are the responsibility of the Home Office and are enforced by the fire authorities in general.

Fire precautions are required to be covered by training staff in the following:

- The means of detection and giving warning in case of fire.
- The means of escape.
- The means of fighting fire.
- The training of staff in fire safety.

The Fire Regulations also include a requirement to undertake an assessment of the fire risks, which should cover both the risk of fire occurring and the risk to people in the event of fire. Advice on carrying out a fire risk assessment (which may be carried out as part of the overall health and safety risk assessment for the workplace) is contained in the Home Office/Scottish Executive/Northern Ireland DoE/HSE publication *Fire Safety: An Employer's Guide*.

Matters falling within the scope of HASWA include the storage of flammable materials, the control of flammable vapours, standards of housekeeping, safe systems of work, the control of sources of ignition and the provision of appropriate training. These precautions are enforced by inspectors from the Health and Safety Executive (HSE) or the local authority.

Between them, the Fire Regulations and the Management of Health and Safety at Work Regulations 1999 SI No. 3242 require employers to:

- Carry out a fire risk assessment of the workplace including making adequate provision for any disabled people with special needs who use or may be present on site.
- Identify the significant findings of the risk assessment and the details of anyone who might be especially at risk in case of fire.
- Provide and maintain such fire precautions as are necessary to safeguard those who use the workplace.
- Provide information, instruction and training to employees about the fire precautions in the workplace.

The Office of the Deputy Prime Minister is currently developing new general fire safety legislation for England and Wales. Their aim is to rationalise and consolidate the many pieces of existing legislation and to provide a risk-based approach to fire safety. The new fire legislation is called the Regulatory Reform (Fire Safety) Order and it is due to come into force in 2006. The following websites provide guidance and links on fire and emergency requirements: www.hse.gov.uk; www.homeoffice.gov.uk; www.mi5.gov.uk.

Induction training is well worth the time spent on its planning and delivery, even in small and medium-sized enterprises. Guidance and advice from multidisciplinary sources is particularly useful so as to cover all the essentials ranging from technical aspects of the job through to general health and welfare issues that affect everyone.

Records of induction training should be kept as evidence that it has taken place. The recruitment plan should also include a clear protocol as to the keeping of records of all applications, in line with the requirements of data protection law and related best practice guidance.

It is worth remembering that internal transfers or internally promoted employees may require health assessment for the new post as well as induction training for their new role. There are also certain situations that require special attention, such as the employment of young people, those returning to work after sickness absence or sabbaticals, people who have special health considerations to be taken into account, and people who have workplace adjustments that may need to be checked and reviewed for appropriate compliance.

Preparing to recruit

There is no legal obligation on employers to advertise vacant posts to which they hope to appoint, but it can be difficult for employers to show that they are following good practice in promoting equal opportunities at work if they do not advertise appropriately. For example, if a particular element of the local or national population is under-represented within the workplace currently, efforts should be made to give such people the chance to be considered for appointment. It may also be that the workforce overall appears at one level to match the local demography, whereas closer examination of the data could reveal that particular groups of people are under-represented at more senior levels.

Generally the minimum requirement of good practice is that posts should be advertised internally, but employers must bear in mind the need to ensure, as previously mentioned, that the spread of people is fairly represented at each level within the organisation. A company policy that has an adverse effect on one group of people who are protected from discriminatory practices by law can be held to be indirect discrimination. So internal advertising, while justifiable in many cases, can carry with it an inherent risk of recruiting externally at lower levels only and so could lead to claims of indirect discrimination. The internal/external advertising question should be a considered choice in each case, rather than a norm.

So the obligations on employers to comply with anti-discrimination and equal opportunities legislation begin at the point of advertisement planning. The wording of the advertisement is important. Careless wording of the post, the person

Job description. Person specification. Risk assessment.
Occupational health, human resources, and health and safety alerts.
Define special considerations: use of equipment, driving licences, criminal record checks, vaccinations, etc.
Advertising: images, wording, compliance and circulation.
Applications: define information required of applicants and method. Invite requests for adjustments to meet disability needs.
Interview and selection: fair process and reasonable adjustments accommodated and communicated.
Occupational health clearance, advice pointers, suggested workplace/practice adjustments, risk assessment review.
Checks: references, identity, qualifications, licences, criminal record checks (as applicable), clearance to work in UK.
Offer of employment – if applicable, conditional offer.
Issue terms and conditions of employment, handbooks, policies, etc.
Acceptance by employee.
Training and induction.

Fig. 1.1 Recruitment checklist.

specification criteria given, and even the method of application can lead to major problems. The good news is that this pre-planning investment in careful consideration can provide a template or checklist (Fig. 1.1) that will really help to avoid potentially costly and much more time-consuming problems that might otherwise emerge. There is now comprehensive and very wide-ranging anti-discrimination legislation in place in the UK, with more on the way to cover the outlawing of age discrimination from October 2006. Key anti-discrimination legislation to be taken into account in the preparation of and throughout the recruitment and appointment include:

- The Equal Pay Act 1970
- The Sex Discrimination Acts 1975 and 1986
- The Race Relations Act 1976 and the Race Relations (Amendment) Act 2000
- The Disability Discrimination Act 1995
- The Employment Equality (Religion or Belief) Regulations 2003 SI No. 1660
- The Employment Equality (Sexual Orientation) Regulations 2003 SI No. 1661
- The Employment Equality (Age) Regulations 2006 SI No. 1031

Job descriptions

Having taken due account of the legal standards required, the prudent employer's next step in the recruitment process will be the preparation of the job description.

This should summarise the main duties and responsibilities of the post, give details of accountability, and make mention of the need for change and flexibility. A future change clause stating words along the following lines might be a sensible standard wording:

'This is an outline summary of the key duties of the post/job as currently required. The nature of the business requires flexibility and change to skills and duties over time. Job descriptions will need to be reviewed and revised so as to ensure they relate to the job actually being performed, or to review and incorporate changes expected.

The review procedure is carried out jointly by employees and management. Staff are expected to cooperate fully in consultation discussions with management regarding changes to duties. It is the company's aim to reach agreement on reasonable changes, but if agreement is not possible the company reserves the right to give notice of changes it requires to be implemented to a job description after consultation with the employee.'

If the job is likely to require particular skills such as driving, this should be specified, including the type of licence required. If the nature of the post is such that mobility is a factor then this too should be stated in the job description. It is also important to state any requirements for travel or foreign postings. It is not likely to be helpful, however, simply to make these kinds of clauses standard in job descriptions unless they are genuinely likely to feature as a part of the duties.

Using the job description as the basis for an objective specification follows on next. This should enable the skills, qualifications, experience and characteristics to be drawn up. Often, within those specifications, a minimum level and a desirable level will be set. Care needs to be taken to ensure that desirable attributes are objective requirements so as not to fall foul of the law.

The job description will serve as the key source of information from the prospective employer to the occupational health adviser who is assessing candidates. Without clear information and plain language describing the main duties of the post, health assessment will not be able to be comprehensive. Occupational health will also provide suggestions as to any adjustments that the employer might consider making to the workplace and working conditions relative to the health needs of the individual. This guidance is reliant on good information via job descriptions and person specifications, which will enable proper risk assessment and enable occupational health to give out the best advice in this respect.

Advertising

Whatever the minimum requirements expected of applicants, advertisements should state this. If there are particular health or related physical criteria that genuinely apply to all applicants for the post being advertised, it is wise to consider and risk assess these in general with an occupational health adviser at the very start of the recruitment exercise.

It is unlawful to word recruitment advertisements in a discriminatory manner. It was not so long ago that job adverts would regularly be seen looking for a 'Girl Friday', which would today render both the advertising publishers and the prospective employer in danger of legal action. But employment rights change and develop rapidly. Some employers advertise seeking a specific age range that may favour the younger applicant, but advertisements can also, by seeking experience that is not an objective requirement, result in discrimination against younger workers. With the Employment Equality (Age) Regulations 2006 in force from October 2006, legal challenges to hitherto accepted recruitment criteria can be expected in this area.

Care must be taken with all the material provided in advertising the post. Wording is crucial but so too are the images presented in the advert itself and in any accompanying literature. Good practice will be to ensure the provision of recruitment material in various formats: in other languages to address and encourage racial balance, in large print or Braille, and on computer email or disk to enable and encourage sight- or hearing-disabled applicants.

Many organisations have a standard advertisement layout, which may include, for example, statements concerning the organisation's aims in equal opportunities and treatment. These can be positive statements, as intended by the wording, but any promises reasonably inferred from them will also need to be honoured. For example, an employer's statement that it will offer an interview to any disabled

Case law

For the National Air Traffic Service and Ben Sargeaunt-Thomson,[1] a deal of upset and cost could perhaps have been avoided if a pre-planned recruitment protocol had been in use by the multidisciplinary team from the start. Mr Sargeaunt-Thomson had a long-standing ambition to become an air traffic controller. He passed all the required entry tests and came through the interview selection process with flying colours despite stiff competition. He was offered his dream job subject to a satisfactory health assessment. At that stage his job offer was justifiably withdrawn on the grounds that no suitable workstation, including visual display screen equipment, could be adapted to take account of his height. At 6 feet 10 inches, Sargeaunt-Thomson argued that NATS recruitment policy was discriminatory as more men than women are likely to be tall. Despite his having gone on to be appointed with Eurocontrol as a trainee with the air traffic control service in Luxembourg, where his workstation could be adapted for his height, the tribunal did not support his claim. The desks at NATS are currently for use by people who are between 5 ft and 6 ft 1 in tall, and the Southampton Employment tribunal accepted that in this particular case the problem could lead to an adverse effect on the ability to do the job safely. Although NATS has reportedly stated that it is pleased not to have been found to have a discriminatory policy, and Mr Sargeaunt-Thomson has found an alternative post, both parties might be wishing that the height criterion had been properly thought through and brought to the attention of potential applicants at the outset. Instead a lengthy recruitment and selection process of over two years took place, disappointment was caused to an individual, and legal action resulted over an issue that could perhaps have been addressed at the initial stages of planned recruitment by a multidisciplinary team.

applicant may not be wise unless that promise can really be met. One that states that an interview will be offered to any disabled candidate who meets the qualification criteria for the post may be a more prudent approach.

Applications

Some employers seek applications by curriculum vitae, letter, on line methods or paper application form. An advantage of using application forms is the standardisation of information required of each and every candidate, making fair comparison easier and ensuring that all necessary information is given. Where the employer does not use application forms, consideration should be given to asking applicants to ensure that they give precise and particular information on specified matters required by the company in their CV submissions. It is important good practice to invite applicants to advise of any special needs they would like to be considered so as to enable the organisation to ensure that no applicant is unfairly disadvantaged on account of disability. A written notice to this effect should be sent to all applicants. It is worth bearing in mind that many people who have disabilities would in no way regard themselves as suffering from ill health. However, where all applicants have been invited to advise of any special needs they have to accommodate their disability, but then fail to do so, they could have some difficulty in later trying to prove that a prospective employer knew or ought to have known of their disability.

The Disability Discrimination Act 1995 (DDA) requires that employers ensure they do not treat disabled people less favourably than others during the recruitment process. Along with the Act itself, there is a Code of Practice, which is a useful guide as to suggested good standards in employment. The legal duty to make reasonable adjustments applies at the recruitment stage and not just to those appointed to take up employment. This is at variance with some other forms of anti-discrimination legislation, which generally requires that all applicants be treated equally. The disability discrimination legislation requires that employers and prospective employers make arrangements where possible to ensure that disabled people are not placed at a disadvantage to non-disabled people. Under section 4 of the DDA it is unlawful to discriminate against a disabled job applicant:

- in the arrangements made for determining to whom employment should be offered, s.4(1)(a), or
- in the terms on which employment is offered, s.4(1)(b), or
- by refusing to offer, or deliberately not offering, the disabled person employment, s.4(1)(c).

Applicants should be encouraged to provide relevant information about their health and personal details. Employers are well advised to make clear that their purpose in seeking such information is to enable proper monitoring and compliance with equality of treatment and opportunity in the workplace. Many people are sensitive to providing information about their gender, marital status, ethnic origins, nationality or any disability for a variety of understandable reasons. Such concerns can be taken on board and positively addressed in the recruitment process. For example, people can be informed at the time the request is made by the employer that the details they provide will be treated as confidential in accordance with data protection standards – see Chapter 2. The law requires that only necessary and relevant information is sought and appropriately retained. It is good practice to consider storing medical information separately, with occupational health if this service is available. If not, then all confidential information must be kept securely to ensure proper privacy.

Information that comes to the attention of the employer must be fairly and properly used. It is worth bearing in mind that many people have a health matter that might now come under the definition of a disability within the meaning of the DDA but which they do not consider means that they are disabled. The DDA defines a disability as

> 'a physical or mental impairment which has a substantial and long term adverse effect on his or her ability to carry out normal day to day activities.'

For many responsible employers a significant problem arises because job applicants and employees do not tell them of any health concerns relevant to the job. They may choose not to do so for fear of discrimination on disclosure of the information or they may not regard the matter as relevant to their working life. An employer, or prospective employer, is obliged to make reasonable adjustments when he knows or ought reasonably to know about a person's disability. If an employer has encouraged applicants from the start and throughout the recruitment process to give information about health matters relevant to the job, then this will usually form a good basis for defending against claims should the applicant later be found to have not given information that was reasonably requested.

Selection

The interview process, together with any selection tests that are used, needs to be planned with care and advice from human resources and occupational health so as to check for fairness and legal compliance. Adjustments should be made where possible to accommodate the needs of applicants. This is important throughout the interview and selection process. The choice of venue, for example, must be accessible to all candidates. If aptitude or other testing is used, any special health-related needs of candidates should be accommodated where possible. Any equipment, printed materials, etc. should be checked to ensure that disabled people are not disadvantaged, e.g. by using enlarged print for those with sight problems, by using written communications for those with hearing problems, and by providing workstation adaptations for those with mobility needs. Employers must now consider reasonable adjustments for disabled people throughout the recruitment and selection process as well as during their employment, should the need arise. A failure to consider reasonable adjustments in these circumstances means an employer will usually not be able to use the so called 'justification' defence, which ceased to be lawful in 2004 save for in particular circumstances.

All evaluations, including interview notes and any scorings, must be fairly and objectively considered. Records should be kept so as to deal with queries or challenges. Many people value some individual feedback being given to them as to why their application has not been successful. When this is provided, even disappointing news is often accepted as fair and non-discriminatory.

Offers of employment

If a job offer is made and accepted then a legal contract exists between the parties from that point. It is a misconception that can lead to costly litigation to assume that the employment contract only comes into force when the employee takes up employment and/or when the written terms and conditions of employment have been signed by the parties. Each element of the recruitment process can contribute to the employment contract, including advertisements, job descriptions, and job offers made verbally or in writing.

Some employers make job offers conditional upon their receiving satisfactory health reports and/or positive references. Any retraction of a job offer made, whether conditional or not, could lead to legal challenge. Claims could arise, for example, for breach of contract and result in an award to cover the notice period that ought to have been expected in the position. More costly still is the potential claim of discrimination on the grounds of race, sex, disability, religious belief, sexual orientation or age. There is no upper limit on the award levels tribunals can make in discrimination cases.

When a job offer is made, whether verbally or in writing, that is conditional upon a satisfactory health report, it is prudent to advise the prospective employee not to resign their current post until a job offer is confirmed to them in writing. This will be after all screenings for references and health have taken place. It is much more likely that an individual will take legal action if they have resigned from a substantive position on the strength of a perceived job offer that is then withdrawn. If an applicant is found to have a cause for concern about their health revealed by an occupational health assessment, this is likely to be an issue for that person. Aside from disappointment in not being successful in their job application, it is likely also to be a sensitive and possibly anxious time. Best practice would be to ensure that all occupational health matters have been clarified with the individual before job offers are made, in the best interests of all concerned.

The government and the Disability Rights Commission have produced a number of codes of practice, explaining legal rights and requirements under the Disability Discrimination Act 1995. These Codes are practical guidance rather than statutory requirements or regulations. However, courts and tribunals must take them into account as evidence of good practice and of possible acts of discriminatory practice.

Section 7 of the Code of Practice for the elimination of discrimination against disabled people[2] provides useful examples and guidance as to the full range of recruitment issues. Helpful pointers are provided to assist employers in developing job descriptions and person specifications that are fair, objective, relevant to

Case law

In *Paul* v. *National Probation Service* [2004] IRLR 190, the occupational health adviser said that he was not fit to supervise people on probation one day per week because he was chronically depressed. However, the person who was given the job was eased into it slowly with supervision and assistance that could have been given to Mr Paul. In any event, the employer was found to have been wrong not to have taken a report from a psychiatrist as to Mr Paul's fitness for the job.

In *Williams* v. *Channel 5 Engineering Services Ltd*, IDS Brief 609/13, the employer failed to seek information about disability in the job application process and so, even though the person who interviewed Mr Williams was told that he was deaf, the information did not get taken on board when the training for the job began. As a result, Channel 5 Engineering was found to have discriminated against Mr Williams in failing to put in place the reasonable adjustments necessary for him to complete the training and in so doing to have treated him less favourably because of his disability.

Adjustments must be reasonable and be directly related to the job. This is exampled well in the case of *Kenny* v. *Hampshire Constabulary* [1999] IRLR 76. Here it was held that the employer was not obliged to provide a carer to accompany Ms Kenny to the lavatory and assist her as was required because of the disability she suffered as a result of cerebral palsy.

In *Murray* v. *Excel Airways Ltd* (2001) ET Case No. 2303006/0, the applicant was offered a position as cabin crew subject to satisfactory references and medical screening. When the company received her medical questionnaire information, they rescinded their offer of employment on the grounds of medical advice they had received. A GP report also obtained noted that Ms Murray had problems in managing her diet and insulin. This, coupled with the nature of the duties, which could present problems with regular meal breaks, meeting dietary requirements and health and safety of passengers in an emergency, led to their considered decision that they could not offer her the post. The tribunal agreed with Excel Airways. Genuine health and safety issues will take precedence over all other considerations in making adjustments and accommodating health concerns at work.

In *Plimley* v. *Newcastle College* (1999) ET Case No. 6402533/99, the tribunal found that Ms Plimley had not been discriminated against by the college when the college occupational health doctor decided she was not fit to do the job as she might be likely to suffer from stress-related health problems. She had applied for vacancies in a department that was known to work under pressure. On the medical questionnaire she noted that she suffered from high blood pressure and was taking medication usually prescribed for depressive conditions. The case demonstrates the value of the occupational health department being told the details of the job to enable them to advise; of risk assessment programmes being completed; and of objective evaluation being properly conducted by the recruitment team.

the duties of the post and non-discriminatory. Sound advice is provided to show the dangers of too widely set job requirements or careless wording that could lead to the courts. It suggests, for example, avoidance of the stipulation that applicants need to be 'active and energetic' when the nature of the job is essentially sedentary. It cautions against blanket exclusions and gives a good example of this in a situation where an employer suggests that persons who suffer from epilepsy will not be considered for driving jobs. In fact, jobs that require only an ordinary driving licence need not necessarily exclude those who have not suffered an epileptic episode within the period specified by the DVLA, and who are therefore entitled to hold a driver's licence and can obtain insurance cover.

Occupational health perspectives

What is occupational health?

Occupational health is not a new medical discipline, but has been around in one form or another for several hundred years. The father of occupational medicine is claimed to be Dr Ramazzini, who published the first edition of his most famous book, the *De Morbis Artificum Diatriba* (Diseases of Workers) in 1700 – the first comprehensive work on occupational diseases, outlining the health hazards of irritating chemicals, dust, metals, and other abrasive agents encountered by workers in 52 occupations. Previously occupational health was called industrial medicine but with the changing world, increasing technology, the advent of computers and more service industries it was changed in the early 1950s to occupational health, and the term 'workplace health management' is often used today to describe its remit.

The twelfth session of the joint International Labor Organization/WHO Committee on Occupational Health, Geneva 1995, set out the objectives of an occupational health programme as follows:

- To maintain and promote workers' health and working capacity.
- To improve the working environment and make it more conducive to safety and health.
- To develop work organisation and the working culture to support health and safety, and promote a positive social climate and smooth operation, which can also enhance productivity.

With these objectives in mind it is important to fit the right person to the job but also to make sure that the job fits the person, as this is the beginning of maintaining the worker's health and working capacity. Part of management and human resources responsibility is to ensure that the right person is employed, taking into account the job specification and the qualifications and experience of the applicants. Occupational health and health and safety personnel support this by advising on aspects of the job that may affect the health of the individual, and by advising management on the health of the individual, both mental and physical. Because of this, there are specialised professionals in this field, and occupational health and safety may consist of:

- occupational health physicians
- occupational health nurses
- occupational hygienists

- ergonomists
- health and safety personnel
- physiotherapists
- occupational psychologists

The professional codes of ethics that cover occupational health physicians and nurses, and certain other qualified professionals such as chartered physiotherapists and psychologists, help to safeguard the confidential medical information they receive from individual workers and so restrict the type of information that can be given to employers and others (see Appendix 1).

Risk assessments

Good employment practice requires prospective employees to be given a job description as part of their contract of employment. Health and safety law requires that a risk assessment be undertaken to identify the hazards and quantify the risks that a worker may be exposed to in the course of their work. The Management of Health and Safety at Work Regulations 1999 SI No. 3242 require employers to undertake a suitable and sufficient risk assessment of the workplace, which means assessing not just the building and all that is in it, but also the risks of each person's job or role within the organisation, no matter where they are working. This can then provide a basis from which a health assessment can be made. When it is known what is required of the job, where it is to take place and what hazards the employee will be exposed to, criteria can be decided against which an assessment of a person's fitness to undertake that role can be decided.

Today there are big differences in health risks depending on the demand of the task or job, but the general laws protecting health and safety apply in all cases. There is some more specific legislation applied in specialist areas, such as chemicals and substances that come under specific legislation, including the Control of Substances Hazardous to Health Regulations 2002 SI No. 2677 (as amended), the Control of Asbestos at Work Regulations 2002 SI No. 2675, and the Control of Noise at Work Regulations 2005 SI No. 1643. These noise regulations came into force in April 2006, with a two-year transitional period for the music and entertainment industry until 6 April 2008. These will be dealt with in more detail in Chapter 3.

Risk assessment is the responsibility of the employer to undertake, and this responsibility can be, and usually is, devolved to the managers or specialists of particular areas of work. Today, as part of quality control systems such as clinical governance in health care, risk managers are employed to consider all aspects of risk, and that can include environmental and financial as well as health and safety factors. However, they too devolve risk assessment to local levels of management that should know and understand the hazards and risks of their area of work. The Health and Safety Executive (HSE) define HAZARD as anything that can cause harm (e.g. chemicals, electricity, working from ladders), and RISK as the chance, high or low, that somebody will be harmed by the hazard.[3] This concept of risk

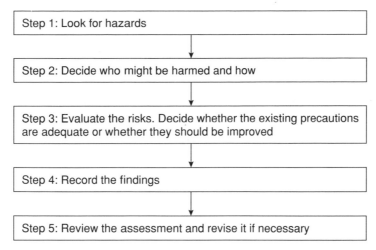

Fig. 1.2   Five steps to risk assessment (HSE 1998)[3].

assessment has alarmed some employers and they have in some instances tried to pass the responsibility on to occupational health, or have avoided getting to grips with their obligations under the legislation. Today the risk assessments records are one of the first things an HSE inspector asks to see when he visits a company, and particularly following an accident or incident reportable under the Reporting of Injuries, Diseases and Dangerous Occurrences Regulations (RIDDOR) 1995 SI No. 3163.

The simplicity or complexity of risk assessments will depend on the work of the company. A large chemical organisation will have complex, multi-layered risk assessments drawn up by highly skilled chemical safety engineers while in other organisations departmental managers, who are confident in their knowledge about their departments activities, are able to undertake risk assessments and will call on occupational health, health and safety, or other professional experts, such as ergonomists, appropriately as the need arises. The basis required for any risk assessment under the Health and Safety at Work etc. Act 1974 and the various pieces of legislation, regulations, codes of practice etc. is the Five Steps to Risk Assessment model shown in Fig. 1.2.

Step 1: Look for hazards

This step requires the risk assessor to have an in-depth knowledge of the workplace and the type of work to be undertaken. Not all workers are on one site; many are peripatetic or work away from a central point, such as delivery drivers, maintenance engineers, postmen, etc. Spending time walking around the workplace, talking with employees and asking questions is one way to identify hazards, but in the case of those not based on site the answer may be to spend a day out with these people, and to ask them and their union representatives what they think are significant hazards. HSE suggests that the trivia should be ignored and significant

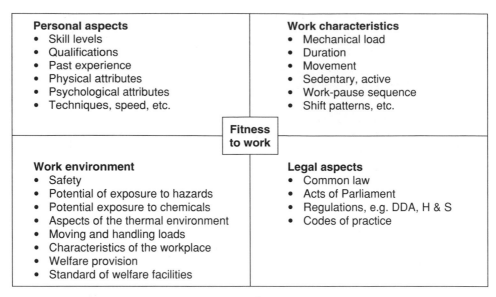

Personal aspects	Work characteristics
• Skill levels	• Mechanical load
• Qualifications	• Duration
• Past experience	• Movement
• Physical attributes	• Sedentary, active
• Psychological attributes	• Work-pause sequence
• Techniques, speed, etc.	• Shift patterns, etc.
Work environment	**Legal aspects**
• Safety	• Common law
• Potential of exposure to hazards	• Acts of Parliament
• Potential exposure to chemicals	• Regulations, e.g. DDA, H & S
• Aspects of the thermal environment	• Codes of practice
• Moving and handling loads	
• Characteristics of the workplace	
• Welfare provision	
• Standard of welfare facilities	

Fitness to work

Fig. 1.3 Fit for work model (Harriss et al., 2002)[4].

hazards concentrated on: by 'significant' they mean hazards that may result in serious harm to the individual or which may affect several people. One good key to identifying hazards is to look under the headings in the work environment and view these along with the work characteristics in Fig. 1.3.

Step 2: Decide who might be harmed and how

The important aspects of this step are those people you may not necessarily have thought about: young workers, expectant mothers, other vulnerable people, or even the general public if you think of such things as building scaffolding or public events. This may lead you to consider that there are some jobs that cannot be undertaken by certain groups, but care must be taken here, and if necessary advice sought, as legislation such as the Disability Discrimination Act 1995 may come into play. It is worth remembering that risk assessments are statutorily required to be carried out for pregnant workers.

Step 3: Evaluate the risks

Some hazards have to be controlled in certain ways according to specific legislation or industry standards, but the majority have to be decided at a local workplace level. It is not always possible to get rid of the hazard but it must always be identified and made known to workers, and its risk mitigated to the lowest risk level practicably possible. Here we quote the example of the sea. It is a natural phenomenon and it does not become a danger until people interact with it, whether for work or pleasure. When consideration is given to all the things that go on by, in, over and under the sea, and the risk factors involved, it presents quite a significant hazard. We cannot get rid of it, nor would we want to, as it is extremely important to life and to our existence. However, we do need to control our inter-action with it in a number of ways, depending on the activity. Some, of course, are controlled by health and safety rules, such fishing, sailing, leisure sports, etc.

Once the risks are evaluated as high, medium or low, they should be reduced to as low as is practicably possible using appropriate measures, including those required by statute. Good practice measures, in addition, will ensure that new employees are suitable for the job and that they have the right health protection at work from the outset. In the case study below, a university demonstrates how it has used the risk assessment process to identify the health assessment and surveillance needs of its employees.

Case study

A university employs some 7500 staff and has a similar number of PhD students and researchers, many of whom are involved in specialist research that involves exposure to known respiratory sensitisers and asthmagens.

The department that is to employ the student or researcher is required to complete an individual risk assessment in relation to the specific research they will be undertaking. On receipt of this assessment by the occupational health service, each individual is required to complete a questionnaire outlining any relevant past medical history and their experience of work in this field. A baseline pre-placement health screen, including spirometry, is then performed on those individuals who are identified as working with known respiratory sensitisers or asthmagens. On completion of this baseline screening, a further three appointments are made for continued screening throughout the succeeding 12-month period in line with Health and Safety Executive guidelines.

To support and strengthen the screening programme, a leaflet, 'Prevention of Sensitisation in Research', has been devised by the occupational health department and is given to every new employee who will be working with the sensitisers or asthmagens. The leaflet provides information on the need for prevention, control of sensitisers and asthmagens, and health surveillance of those individuals working with these sensitisers and asthmagens.

Step 4: Record the findings

This will be dealt with in more depth in Chapter 2, but suffice it to say at this stage that keeping a written record for future reference and for legal purposes is essential. Health surveillance and COSHH risk assessment records should be kept for at least 40 years.

Step 5: Review

Periodic reassessment is important and will help with ensuring that health and safety is kept at the forefront of managers' and workers' minds, and that everything is working effectively and at current best practice standards. Changes to the workplace, equipment or new procedures will all require the risk assessment to be reviewed.

For examples of how to undertake simple risk assessments, see Figs 1.4 and 1.5.

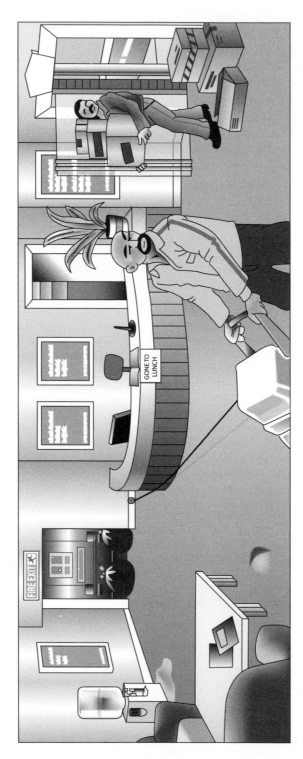

Fig. 1.4 Workplace entrance.

Fig. 1.4 Workplace entrance. There are six hazards in this picture. See if you can identify them and consider who they might harm and how. Then consider how you could remove the hazards or reduce the risk of their causing harm. Check with the table below to see if your risk assessment concurs. This fulfils the first three steps of the risk assessment. Record your findings in a suitable manner, such as the chart below, and then plan review dates.

Step 1 *Identify the hazard*	Step 2 *Decide who might be harmed and how*	Step 3 *Evaluate risks and put in place measures to reduce the risks*
Company entrance unmanned.	This is a security risk and allows anyone to enter the building. No supervision of contractors or deliveries.	Level of risk will depend on where the company is and what it does. Reducing the risk could be quite simple – having a key pad on the door for workers and a bell for visitors.
Manual handling of boxes, and the individual doing this unable to see where he is going.	Risk of slips, trips and falls to the individual or to others he may encounter. Risk of musculoskeletal disorders such as low back pain.	Provide a sack barrow, to minimise manual handling. Provide information and training for safe handling.
Storage blocking both entrances/ fire exits.	A danger to all people who are in the building in the event of a fire or a power cut.	Provide safe storage areas, and information and training about keeping entrances and exits clear at all times.
Electrical wires across the floor.	A hazard to people walking across the area.	Cleaning areas should be cordoned off and signposted while cleaning is in progress; operatives need information and training on correct procedures.
Torn carpet.	Worn and uneven floors are a trip hazard, especially in a public area.	Repair carpet with suitable tape. Inspect public areas regularly. Identify personnel responsible for the area.
Leaking water cooler.	At risk of both an electrical accident and slips or falls.	Sign indicating who to report faults to. Regular maintenance contract. Temporary hazard sign until repaired.

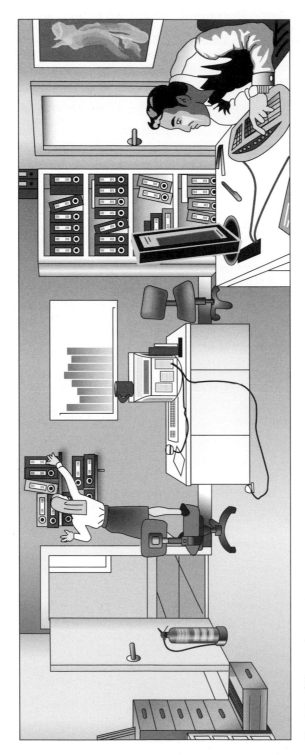

Fig. 1.5   Office environment.

Fig. 1.5 Office environment. There are seven hazards in this picture. See if you can identify them and consider who they might harm and how. Then consider how you could remove the hazards or reduce the risk of their causing harm. Check with the table below to see if your risk assessment concurs. This fulfils the first three steps of the risk assessment. Record your findings in a suitable manner, such as the chart below, and then plan review dates.

Step 1 *Identify the hazard*	Step 2 *Decide who might be harmed and how*	Step 3 *Evaluate risks and put in place measures to reduce the risks*
Poor posture at computer.	Musculoskeletal disorders such as work-related upper limb disorders and back ache.	This needs addressing to prevent ill health and sickness absence. Provide information training for use of display screen equipment (DSE) and undertake a DSE workstation risk assessment.
Door propped open with fire extinguisher.	This is a trip hazard; anyone coming into the office could fall over it. If the door is a fire door, it should be kept shut.	Check the status of the door and whether it needs to be shut for fire prevention purposes; if not, then provide a wooden door wedge. If it is a fire door and the office is too warm, check heating and ventilation with maintenance department. Provide a fan to circulate air.
Filing cabinet drawer open.	Trip hazard to all who use the office.	Information and training to shut filing cabinet drawers after use. Always make sure filing cabinet drawers are well balanced with heaviest things at the bottom.
Using a chair (especially one on castors) to reach heights.	High risk of falling and injury.	Provide office kick stool for reaching heights. Provide suitable storage at a lower level that is easily reachable.
Mug on top of computer.	Liquids and electricity do not mix.	Provide information and training on handling electrical equipment.
Electrical wires across the floor.	A hazard to people walking around the office.	Provide suitable covers for trailing leads from desks and other electrical equipment.
Broken chair.	Someone may sit on this and receive an injury or musculoskeletal problems.	Provide a safe system for labelling, removing and reporting broken equipment.

Health assessment

Health assessment for fitness to undertake a job also has a long history originating from the times when young men were required to undertake tests of endurance for their tribal initiation as warriors.[4] Of course, today this would contravene all sorts of legislation in the UK. Before even getting to the situation of assessing the health of individuals and their suitability for employment in a given post there are a host of rules and regulations to be considered, not to mention a few myths to be dispelled. There are many variables to consider when employing people. Harriss *et al.*'s Fitness to Work Framework of Assessment (Fig. 1.3) is a useful tool for helping to ensure that assessment is comprehensive, equitable and transparent.

Assessing the skill levels of workers is the job of management, but skills can be impaired by underlying physical or mental health problems. Workers may be aware of this and may not disclose this in pre-employment job applications or at interview. It is believed that the confidential nature of occupational health helps to overcome this dilemma, but this will depend on the confidence the organisation displays in the occupational health service as well as the system used for health assessment. Job applicants may not see the relevance of disclosing personal medical information, or they may not fully understand the implications of their medical condition. Much will depend on the nature of the enquiry, whether or not it is specifically job related, and the system used to acquire the information. The existing political climate also has a bearing, in terms of whether there is high or low unemployment. If an applicant is likely to be unemployed or is in competition with others then he may feel compelled to take part in the process,[5] or it may be that he withholds vital information about his mental or physical condition.

In order to be able to make professional, evidence-based decisions on the mental and physical suitability of a prospective employee for a particular job, the occupational health practitioner needs to be thoroughly aware of the job requirements and any risks or health hazards within the duties relative to the individual.

Case study

A qualified and experienced occupational health nurse was employed by a company. The job was peripatetic and involved her visiting other branches of the organisation, so a valid driving licence was required, which she possessed. Once she was employed, the nurse did not seem to be making regular visits to the branches and was often late for appointments. The branch managers with whom she had booked appointments complained about this and the infrequency of the visits. The nurse said that it was because of the poor bus service from the village where she lived and that she preferred to travel by public transport rather than use her car. Her line manager investigated the bus timetables and found that the nurse had not been entirely truthful about the bus times and so tackled her on this, and the nurse agreed to make more effort with her visits in future. Shortly after this she had a serious car accident while en route to one of her appointments.

It subsequently transpired that the nurse suffered from epilepsy and diabetes, and had not declared either of these conditions on her health declaration form as she was concerned that she would not get the job. As she had a valid driving licence and her epilepsy was under control, this need not have prevented her from being employed. The occupational health service would have said she was 'fit for employment with certain provisos' and would have explained these, and then her manager would have been able to offer more support with regard to the frequency and timing of the visits. This might have prevented an accident and the nurse losing her job.

However, for evidence-based practice it is important to note Whitaker and Aw's 1995 research,[6] which concluded that there are limitations in the health assessment process's ability to detect clinical conditions and to predict the health status of employees once they are employed.

Methods of health assessment

Once the risk assessment has been carried out for the relevant workplace and the work to be undertaken within that workplace, it is possible for the occupational health service, together with other stakeholders such as managers, human resources, unions, etc. to devise and approve a suitable method of health assessment. This should be clearly laid out in a suitable occupational health policy. Rantanen states that 'mechanistic health examinations or screening without clearly defined occupational health objectives are not ethically justified'.[7]

Except where there are other legal implications, such as for working with ionising radiation or specific substances, diving, etc. (see Chapter 3), the usual assessments are made initially by paper or remote screening using a questionnaire. This acts as a filter for determining whether a follow-up assessment by an occupational health nurse or doctor is required, depending on what the applicant has declared on the form.

Questionnaire design

Designing suitable health declaration questionnaires can be a problem, and there are certain factors that need to be considered. It is important to remember that questionnaires should only collect as much information as is necessary to fulfil the aims of the inquiry. Personal data should be 'adequate, relevant and not excessive' in relation to the purpose, or purposes, for which they are processed'.[8] Medical jargon should be avoided at all costs; in other words, the questionnaire should be comprehensible and 'user friendly'. After extensive research, Whitaker & Aw produced a suitable pre-employment health declaration form for health care workers,[6] and this can be downloaded from the Department of Health website: www.dh.gov.uk. (see Appendix 2). Although is it designed specifically for health workers, it does provide a good basis from which to adapt a suitable questionnaire for other employments.

Handling the questionnaire

There are many methods of handling the questionnaire in practice, and much is said about the ethical and legal issues. Firstly, at what stage will the questionnaire be completed? Should this be before interview, at interview or at the time of the job offer? The legal issue is that once a job offer has been made a contract exists, unless perhaps it is specified that it is subject to health clearance and that the applicant should not resign from his present employment before the clearance is given. Prospective employees should be informed of the company's procedures, and be told who will handle and see the completed questionnaire. The Faculty of Occupational Medicine (FOM) states that personnel staff are not qualified to interpret medical data, but it is apparent that certain large organisations do use this system as an initial filter and that those health declaration questionnaires may not be confidential to occupational health.

The occupational health professions would recommend that questionnaires are returned to the occupational health department under separate cover, or today in some instances in the form of secure emails, in order that the contents remain confidential, with the hope that prospective employees will trust the confidential nature of the medical and nursing professions and therefore complete the form with openness and trust. Recent straw polls at employment and educational events indicate that people are sometimes not entirely honest when completing these forms, so there is probably a need for further research into this particular area.

Fit for work?

According to company occupational health policy, and based on the risk assessment for the particular job, the occupational health practitioner makes a professional judgement on the fitness of the applicant for the post. Research has shown that the majority of people prove to be fit for employment,[7] and management can be informed of this clearance accordingly. For those not found suitable at this stage, it may be necessary to attend for a health assessment interview by an occupational health nurse or doctor.

> 'A health assessment is a one to one interaction between a client (the employee or prospective employee) and an occupational health professional, usually a doctor or a nurse, for the purposes of assessing the physical and/or mental health status of a client.' (Thornbory 1994)[9]

Local policy and professional knowledge and experience will determine who undertakes the health assessment. The FOM (1999) makes it quite clear that medical examinations should only be undertaken when justified by virtue of:

- risk assessment
- specific standards of mental or physical health
- legal requirements
- health of the applicant impacting on health and safety of others

The occupational health policy should give clear criteria for the nurse as to when and how to refer an applicant to the doctor. If it is the occupational health nurse who carries out the health interview then the health assessment should consist of only those factors identified on the questionnaire as relevant to the post. Research undertaken in 1994 into what occupational health nurses did at pre-employment health assessments indicated that 85% of nurses undertook height, weight, urinalysis and vision screening irrespective of the justification for or relevance of the processes.[8] The Fit for Work: Framework for Assessment,[4] does not go into the 'battery of assessment tools' and there does not appear to be any more recent published research that does deal with this issue. Suffice it to say that assessment is made on each individual applicant according to the advice derived from the framework assessment. According to Schober,[10] assessment of the health needs of the individual is the foundation for all decision-making and problem-solving activities of care. Her work also provides a helpful list of what effective assessment depends on.

Disability discrimination

Care must be taken at this stage as several pieces of legislation are particularly relevant here, not least the Disability Discrimination Act 1995. The Code of Practice, as mentioned previously, gives clear guidance on discrimination in the recruitment of employees, with case studies and examples that illustrate good practice.

Particularly relevant to occupational health are the questions an employer may ask about disability. For example, in order to give sound professional advice to the employer on reasonable adjustments and the safety of employing a person with a disability in a particular post, it is important for the occupational health practitioner to know and understand how the disability affects the client in both the long and short term. It may be that this cannot be ascertained from a questionnaire and the client will need to be called for a health assessment. However, this assessment may only be relevant and fair in relation to how the disability will impact on the health and safety of the client and/or others in the same workplace. Obtaining a history is an important aspect of health assessment, but if the questions being asked are not relevant to the job or to future health status then they should not be asked. On the other hand, asking the client whether any changes or adjustments to the job or work place will be helpful or necessary is a useful and positive enquiry.

It may be that the applicant is found to be fit for the post but that certain modifications or adjustments are required: for example, as in the case of an applicant with a visual impairment, or a progressive illness such as multiple sclerosis (MS). In the case of visual impairment, certain adjustment may be needed to, say, display screen equipment, in which case the advice of a relevant outside body, such as the Royal National Institute for the Blind, or the disability employment adviser (DEA) through Access to Work, could be sought. Alternatively, it may be necessary to obtain more information on the applicant's existing medical condition, and this will require the applicant's permission to contact their GP or hospital consultant for further information. Other legislation would be relevant here too, such as the Data Protection Act 1998, Access to Medical Reports Act 1988 and Access to Health Records Act 1990. Much of this will be covered in the next chapter on records and reports. With certain conditions, such as MS, future predictions are difficult to make; the client may only ever have one episode of visual disturbance,[11] and if there are future episodes help can be sought from the disability employment adviser regarding any necessary workplace adjustments.

Some people will be found to be unsuitable for employment in the position for which they have applied. It should be noted that the person is not necessarily unfit for work, but has been found to be recommended as unfit, or unsuitable from a health and safety perspective, for that particular post. There is no legal requirement for this decision to be made by a doctor, and so who carries this out will depend entirely on the local occupational health policy agreed between the company and the occupational health service. However, the occupational health nurse or doctor must be aware that he or she has to be able to justify the action and that they can demonstrate that it is an evidence-based decision. It would be prudent for the nurse to obtain further medical advice, with the client's permission, from the treating specialist or GP. The occupational health professionals and other medical advisers make their health-related recommendations to management, which in turn enable management to make the decision relating to the employment issues.

References

1. As reported in the *Journal of the Law Society of Scotland*, News, 9 September 2005.
2. Department for Education and Employment (1996) *Code of Practice for the Elimination of Discrimination in the Field of Employment Against Disabled Persons or Those who have had a Disability*. HMSO, London.
3. Health and Safety Executive (1998) *Five Steps to Risk Assessment*. HSE, London.
4. Harriss, A., Murugiah, S. & Thornbory, G. (2002) Assessment of fitness. *Occupational Health* (April), **54** (4), 26–31.
5. Whitaker, S. (2004) Health examinations on new employment: the ethical issues. In: *Practical Ethics in Occupational Health* (eds P. Westerholm, T. Nilstun & J. Ovretviet), 91. Radcliffe, Oxford.
6. Whitaker, S. & Aw, T. C. (1995) Audit of pre-employment assessments by OH departments in the NHS. *Journal of Occupational Medicine*, **45** (2), 75–80.
7. Rantanen, J. (1998) *Ethical and Social Principles in Occupational Health Practice*. Research report 21, Helsinki.
8. Faculty of Occupational Medicine (1999) *Guidance on Ethics for Occupational Physicians*. Faculty of Occupational Medicine, London.
9. Thornbory, G. (1994) Health assessment on occupational health practice. Unpublished MSc dissertation, University of Surrey.
10. Schober, J., Hincliff, S. & Norman, S. (1998) *Nursing Practice and Health Care*, 3rd edn. Arnold, London.
11. Cox, R. (2000) *Fitness for Work: the Medical Aspects*. Oxford University Press, Oxford.

Chapter 2
Records and Reports

Information that employers hold about their workers is usually confidential. Privacy and confidentiality are now protected as such by a raft of legislation. Often the first practical question that arises is to whom is the information confidential? Within that question lie more detailed issues such as which persons are permitted to have all or some knowledge of information held about an individual, and which information is much more restricted? Health and sickness records fall into the latter category, and disclosure rules about this kind of information often lead to uncertainty and even to conflict from time to time.

For medical and nursing professionals, a breach of due confidentiality can lead not only to disciplinary action but also to professional misconduct allegations. They are required to meet the standards of competence, care and conduct prescribed by their professional bodies. Similarly, human resource professionals who are chartered members of their professional body, the Chartered Institute of Personnel and Development (CIPD), must comply with a code of professional conduct.

From time to time, and usually when there is an issue about absence levels or work performance, general management may seek information that could impinge upon patient/client confidentiality. There is now legislation, as well as set professional conduct standards, to ensure that no personal information is disclosed without consent, save in exceptional circumstances. Where these exceptional circumstances may apply, best practice would be to take advice from legal and professional advisers as cases may differ depending on their own facts and circumstances. Based on requisite standards, good practice is that organisations set out their internal protocols to ensure confidentiality and legal compliance generally.

Legal perspectives

The Data Protection Act 1998

This is a key piece of legislation covering all aspects of employment and in particular information about workers' health. The Data Protection Act (DPA) actually came into force in March 2000, with certain provisions at that time being transitional so as to give employers and other organisations time to comply fully with its requirements. As with all legislation, it is time well spent to check for updates and changes from time to time. The Information Commissioner's own website is the most useful starting point for this purpose as well as for more detailed information and guidance on the subject: www.dataprotection.gov.uk, or www.informationcommissioner.gov.uk.

The legislation recognises that the individual has the basic right to expect that personal information will be treated as confidential. That individual, called the 'data subject' in the Act, has the right to choose whether or not to release personal data, to know what happens to the information once it has taken the form of a tangible record, and to be sure that it is correct at any given point in time. As all data kept about people must be accurate and up to date, regular audits and secure erasing or destruction of papers is a good practice requirement. Personal data encompasses all employment records kept on an individual, including expressions of opinion, intentions, plans, assessments, etc. It is a criminal offence to breach the legal requirements of the Act by failing to process information properly and fairly.

An employee has the right, as the data subject, to be given information by the employer about what records are held on any file concerning their employment details. They can ask the employer what information is held about them, who receives it and why it is used, and they can request a copy of the information. The employee is expected to pay a fee for the request being met, and the employer has 40 days in which to respond. It is good practice to have a standard request form, with the fee invoice issued at the same time, provided to anyone making a request covered by this provision. The response form should make it clear how much the fee is, to whom it is to be paid and the payment methods accepted, and it should make clear that the request, and the 40-day response time period, will only begin to be actioned after the formal request with the due payment is received. Fee rates are set to have maximum charge levels depending upon the type of data provided: see the website of the Information Commissioner's office for current fee levels.

If an individual believes that information held on him is untrue or inaccurate, he can ask for it to be corrected or destroyed. If an employer refuses to do so, the courts have jurisdiction to order the employer to take such action as is deemed necessary to protect the employee's position. The employee can claim compensation for damage or distress caused by inaccurate data processing or unauthorised disclosure.

Sensitive data

There are additional restrictions and standards that apply to what the Act calls 'sensitive personal data'. This covers information about an individual's personal circumstances including ethnic or racial origin, political or religious beliefs, trade union membership or affiliation, sexual or marital status, criminal records and, crucially for occupational health purposes, information about a person's physical or mental health. Records like this can only be held with the consent of the individual. This is usually stated in the employment contract.

References are usually given in confidence by a third party for employment or training purposes. In those circumstances confidential references need not usually be disclosed. Where confidential references are to be disclosed, compliance rules that apply to references, as covered in the Act, must be followed.

The Act's principles

The DPA sets this into a solid legal framework within eight principles, which are the cornerstone of data protection in the workplace. The eight principles require that personal data shall be:

- Processed fairly and lawfully.
- Obtained only for specified and lawful purposes.
- Adequate, relevant and not excessive in relation to the purposes for which it is processed.
- Accurate and up to date.
- Not kept for longer than necessary, relative to the purpose for which the data were processed originally.
- Processed in accordance with the rights of the individual.

And personal data shall:

- Have appropriate technical and organisational measures taken to prevent un-authorised or unlawful processing and accidental loss, destruction or damage.
- Only be transferred within the European Economic Area or to countries that have equivalent data protection systems.

The principles relate to the processing of personal data, otherwise known as information. This is an important note: there are sometimes misconceptions that 'data' refers only to computer-held records, but this is not the case. Any information records that are kept in an identifiable filing or retrieval system are covered by the Act. Similarly, 'processing' is not confined to computer processes but is more widely defined to cover collection, storage, organisation, retrieval, alteration, disclosure or destruction. All these principles are applicable to the obtaining, maintenance, transfer and, at the end of their useful life, safe and proper destruction of occupational health records kept on computer or in an identifiable filing system. The Freedom of Information Act 2000 has also added to the DPA's definition of 'personal data'.

Every organisation that stores or uses personal information must notify and register as a named data controller with the Information Commission (IC) as part of the compliance process. This is done directly with the IC and is a simple and straightforward process. There is an annual fee payable, with the notification set up to be completed online. An occupational health company or individual that provides services to a third-party company must complete data notification registration in its own right if it holds any records in its own manual files or computer records. The data protection notification of the client company alone is not sufficient in these circumstances.

Sensitive personal data and when disclosure is permitted

The DPA requires compliance with defined conditions with regard to the processing of sensitive personal information. All health records, including occupational health notes, reports and reasons for sickness and absence, are classified as sensitive personal data under the legislation.

To process sensitive information lawfully there must be compliance with the appropriate conditions. This includes ensuring that:

- The express consent of the data subject has been freely given.
- The processing is necessary to comply with an obligation or legal duty.
- The processing is necessary to protect the vital interests of the data subject or another person, such as disclosure of a medical condition to a doctor in a medical emergency.
- The processing is necessary for or in connection with legal proceedings or in order to exercise a legal right or to obtain legal advice.
- The information is necessary for monitoring equal opportunities and treatment and/or the data held in the personal record data have been made public by the subject for equal opportunities monitoring.
- The processing is necessary in the public interest.

The Employment Practices Code

The Employment Practices Code was issued by the Information Commissioner in 2005 to help to guide and advise employers on best practice in compliance with the Act.

The four-part Code states the need to 'strike a balance between the legitimate expectations of workers that personal information about them will be handled properly and the legitimate interests of employers in deciding how best, within the law, to run their own businesses'. Knowledge and taking account of the Code are essential for occupational health, human resource professionals and management, since it sets out some appropriate standards guidance for dealing with data that go beyond the basic ethical and legal requirements of medical confidentiality.

The Code is not legally binding and nor is it prescriptive, to be followed in each and every situation. Instead it provides a useful guide to the kinds of situations employers can face, good practice examples as to how particular situations might be handled, general policy frameworks and protocol guidance. While the Code has no legal force, it can be used in evidence as to standards of conduct and compliance with legislation. Failure to take account of the Code could be evidence of negligence or breach of data protection requirements. In addition to the Code, there is a quick guide to the Code that is especially useful to smaller employers. Supplementary guidance that may be particularly helpful to larger organisations is also available.

A useful starting point is the definition of a 'worker'. The term is used in its broadest definition in the Act and the Code, and for this purpose workers are:

- All applicants, successful and unsuccessful, past and current.
- Employees, current and leavers.
- Agency staff, current and past.
- Casual staff, current and past.
- Contract staff, current and past.
- Volunteers and work experience placements.

The Code has been produced in four parts covering:

(1) Recruitment and selection.
(2) Employment records.
(3) Monitoring at work.
(4) Workers' health.

The Code recommends how employers can meet their obligations under the Act, explaining the steps that must be taken to ensure that data are stored and accessed under strict conditions and specifying in section 4 how medical records and health information – 'sensitive data' – is to be dealt with. The importance of the worker's needing to give explicit consent on the basis that, as the data subject, he knows what he is consenting to, and how the information given will be used, is clear. The worker must be permitted to refuse consent 'without penalty' and to withdraw consent once given. Good practice would be to ensure that consent should be renewed from time to time, as the Code states that 'blanket consent obtained at the outset of employment cannot always be relied on'.

Sickness and injury records are often mixed with general absence records. The Code suggests that good practice is that they be separated, for example by a computer password. The Code points out that the law may be changed to cover aspects of the way that sickness and injury records are kept. It is worth noting that the Health and Safety Executive has revised its Workplace Accident Book to take account of the confidentiality requirement. In the meantime, best practice is to deal with all sickness and absence records as sensitive data and afford them the relevant degree of security to avoid breaches of privacy or misuse. The Code points out that 'league tables' of sickness absence of individual workers 'should not be published because the intrusion of privacy in doing so would be disproportionate to any managerial benefit'.

The Code repeats the basic principle that managers do not need medical details about individual workers or members of their families. At a practical level, if an employee has explicitly consented to such disclosure this may make absence or claims on an occupational health scheme more understandable to management and may assist all parties. The Code confirms that consent to disclosure in such circumstances should be in writing. Quality and security standards in many organisations require that e-mails and telephone conversations be monitored. The Code points out that if any confidential information is retrieved accidentally the accidental recipient should delete it and keep no record of it. Staff should be informed, through company policy and protocols, that where confidential information might accidentally come to their notice, the recipient is bound by the utmost confidentiality in respect of the acquired knowledge, and must inform management to ensure investigation and deletion of the information. Workers who allege that confidential information has been inappropriately obtained or transmitted must be given the right to raise a complaint and, if necessary, an internal grievance.

The Code can be downloaded in its entirety via the Information Commissioner's website (www.informationcommissioner.gov.uk), while a summarised version is provided below.

The Employment Practices Code: A Checklist

- Employers should be aware that the mere obtaining of health information is intrusive.
- Workers have a legitimate expectation that their employers will respect their privacy with regard to their health information (this is a basic human right under Article 8 of the European Convention on Human Rights, incorporated into the Human Rights Act 1998).
- Collecting and holding health information must be done with a clear purpose and justified by real benefits.
- Company policies must be comprehensively reviewed or written to cover the Act and best practice standards, including express consent.
- Secure record storage protocols must be in place for manual files and computer records, in particular for restricted access sensitive data.
- Record retention and destruction parameters must be set for manual and computer-filed data.
- Manually filed and computer records are to be audited and monitored.

Employers will need to consider their own workplace needs in relation to the Code of Practice recommendations in order to develop their own protocols: an example follows as a guide.

RECORD RETENTION TIME GUIDE – (YEARS)	
Application form	1
References received	1
Medical reports	3
Sickness records	3
Annual leave records	2
Disciplinary sanction	1 from expiry of warning
Summary record of employment	10
Accident or injury	12 from end of employment
Health surveillance records	Up to 50 years

Health records and confidentiality

Records that contain any details about a worker's health, whether kept by occupational health professionals or by management, are considered in law to be 'sensitive data' since they contain health information. Medical records are, in this sense, the property of the individual to whom they relate for the purposes of disclosure. The DPA provides for special rules relating to medical and social work records (Data Protection Act (Subject Access Modification) (Health) Order 2000). That individual's consent must be given, save for in exceptional and defined circumstances as set out in the DPA, before they can be disclosed. There is also other legislation that covers some of the exceptional circumstances where there may be a legal obligation to disclose medical information to a public body: for example, reporting notifiable infectious diseases to public health authorities.[1] Detailed information on the complex area of confidentiality and disclosure obligations is provided in *Occupational Health Law*, by Diana Kloss.[2] The general rule is disclosure only with the express consent of the individual. Where a demand is made, for example by a legal representative, to disclose without such consent, then a court order will be required. Disclosures without consent should only be made after taking legal and professional advice.

Health information and medical records can cover a wide range of issues that occur in the employment situation from routine appointments to telephone or online consultations, emails, results of drug and alcohol tests, vaccinations, industrial injuries, counselling consultations, health questionnaires, medical certificates, medical reports, and any health information required to be kept by legislation or in anticipation of litigation. It is likely that any personal information provided by a worker to an occupational health professional in the course of a consultation could be construed as sensitive health information data, whether this is through a counselling session or the completion of a health questionnaire. Clearly, where fitness to work is assessed in relation to taking up or returning to employment, or in considering reasonable adjustments where the Disability Discrimination Act 1995 applies, personal data of a sensitive nature will be processed.

A health record is defined in the Act as being any record that consists of information relating to the physical or mental health or condition of an individual, and has been made by or on behalf of a health professional in connection with the care of that individual. Health records cover the full range of media by which information can be held on an individual including, for example, scans, X-rays, print-out results, computer records and handwritten notes.

A health record kept under a health surveillance programme is different from a medical record as it should not contain confidential clinical details. These records should be kept as confidential personnel records. The HSE recommends[3] that health surveillance records should contain the following: name, gender, age, address, date of joining present job, record of job(s) involving exposure to hazard(s), date and conclusions of health surveillance procedures. These conclusions can contain assessments made by doctors, nurses, or other suitably qualified or responsible persons, but must not contain clinical information.

The Access to Health Records Act 1990, which gave individuals the right to access their manually held medical records, has now been repealed save for the access to health records of the deceased. Records of living persons now fall within the protection of the Data Protection Act 1998. Subject access rights to health records now follow the Act's provisions, including fee-charging levels. As previously noted, current fee rates and full details of these provisions should be checked via the Information Commissioner's website. Currently a maximum fee of £10.00 can be charged for granting access to health records that are automatically processed. For granting access to manually held records, or a mixture of automated and manual record files, where the subject access is granted by the supply of a copy of the information in permanent form (a printout, paper copy or disk), a maximum fee of £50.00 can be charged. No fee can be charged to someone who simply wants to inspect their own health records.

Health reports

The Access to Medical Reports Act 1988 (AMRA) gives individuals a right of access to medical reports relating to them that are supplied by doctors for employment purposes. An employer may not apply to a medical practitioner or, it follows, to another health professional for such a report without the employee's consent.

Problems as to the legal framework and related obligations can sometimes occur because the legislation is covered today over different Acts, case law decisions and regulations, many of which are complex – quite apart from the difficulty of piecing together the relevant law. The key aspects of the legal standards are as follows:

- A medical report is defined as one prepared by a medical practitioner who is or has been 'responsible for the clinical care of the individual' (Access to Medical Reports Act 1988). It is the case in practice that occupational health specialists and other health professionals, whether or not they have responsibility for the clinical care of the individual, may also write reports for employment purposes. Their obligations are guided but not enforced by the AMRA. The precise legal obligations for these types of medical reports are also covered by the Data Protection Act 1998, together with the health practitioner's own professional standards of conduct and ethical guidelines. In the Access to Health Records Act 1990, a 'health professional' is exampled as being a medical practitioner, dentist, registered nurse, physiotherapist, optician, dietician, clinical psychologist, occupational therapist, speech therapist, etc. The list is not exhaustive but essentially it refers to those professionals who are qualified, registered and bound by a professional code of conduct and ethics.
- Employees have the right of access to medical reports relating to them including those supplied for employment purposes.
- Employers must notify the employee in writing of their intention to apply for a medical report. This can be achieved through its being express in the written terms and conditions of employment, but problems could arise if this is challenged and so our best practice recommendation would be to ensure that the contract of employment covers the point and that written permission from the employee is obtained when the clause is to be exercised. It has been shown by case law testing that when an employee consents to a medical examination that person can be deemed to have given their consent to a report of that examination being disclosed without further consent being required. Again, this is a matter of judgement as to what is best practice and best employment relations standards as well as what meets the minimum legal standards.
- When the employer seeks to obtain consent from the employee, he must advise of the statutory right to refuse to allow a report to be supplied, and to see its contents and to request alterations or amendments before it is supplied.
- Retrospective access is allowed to the subject of a report provided for employment reasons for up to six months from the date when the report was originally provided.

- Access to the full report, or part of it, can be denied to the subject by the doctor if it is reasonably believed that the disclosure might be likely to cause physical or mental harm to the person, or if it involves the disclosure of the identity of a third party without that person's consent.

The employee or prospective employee is entitled to see the report and be given the opportunity to correct any errors before it is supplied to a third party, and to withhold consent to the report being supplied. There are implications for employees to consider should they unreasonably refuse to consent to a medical examination and to the release of a report. Contracts of employment should contain an express wording as to the right to request and require a medical report. The wording of this should be reasonable but must cover the band of situations where a medical report could be necessary rather than be so narrowly restricted to returners from lengthy sickness absence situations.

Case law

The Medical Reports Act 1988 provides that employees are not obliged to disclose medical records to their employer. Disclosure is only possible where the employee has given his or her written consent. However, sick employees who consistently refuse to provide the necessary consent can be fairly dismissed, as the claimant found to her cost in *Elmbridge Housing Trust* v. *O'Donoghue* [2004] EWCA Civ 939 CA. Ms O'Donoghue was absent because of 'stress or depression'. While on sick leave she insisted that her employer communicate with her only through her trade union representative. After seven weeks, her employer requested her to complete a form giving consent to being seen by the employer's occupational health advisers. After considerable delay, and after her employer had extended the deadline for her to do so three times, Ms O'Donoghue returned the form, but she then refused to consent to the occupational health advisers providing a report to the employer. Eventually Ms O'Donoghue did give her full consent, but she then refused to complete a further form that was required by the occupational health advisers. After three months of further wrangling the employer dismissed her on the ground of incapability. A tribunal found that the dismissal was fair, but the EAT overturned the tribunal's decision. The case moved to the Court of Appeal, which held that the tribunal's decision had not been perverse: the employer had shown that Ms O'Donoghue's presence on site was vital, and her employer was entitled to seek to clarify the reason for her absence and to enable a solution to be found. The employer had done all it reasonably could to elicit further medical information and had been hampered by the lack of direct communication with Ms O'Donoghue. They had reasonably and repeatedly extended deadlines to afford the employee the chance to cooperate. Given her consistent refusal to provide her effective consent, the employer had waited for a reasonable period before dismissal. In the circumstances, the employer had acted within the range of reasonable responses open to it and, on the strength of the evidence available, was entitled to conclude that the employee was incapable of fulfilling her employment obligations and she had been fairly dismissed.

In *Hanlon* v. *Kirklees Metropolitan Council and Others* (2004) EAT 0119/04 (IDS Brief 767), the EAT faced the difficulty of reconciling the competing rights to privacy and

Cont.

proper conduct of a legal matter. In this case, the Employment Appeal Tribunal upheld a tribunal's decision to strike out a disability discrimination claim where the employee declined to give consent to disclosure of his medical records on the ground that this would contravene his right to privacy. The tribunal was confirmed as correct in its judgment that the decision with regard to the right to privacy of medical records had to be balanced with the need to release relevant information in order to permit the proper conduct of the litigation.

In *De Keyser Ltd* v. *Wilson* [2001] IRLR 324, a tribunal cited an alleged breach of an employee's human right to privacy as a ground for striking out the employer's notice of appearance. On appeal, the EAT took a different view, holding that a letter of instruction sent to the occupational health specialist appointed by the employer to examine the employee had not infringed Wilson's privacy. None of the information contained in the letter was obtained surreptitiously or given to Wilson in confidence.

In *Dalgleish* v. *Lothian Borders Police Board* [1991] IRLR 422, it was held that employees' names and addresses were confidential and could not be disclosed to third parties.

In *Durant* v. *Financial Services Authority* [2003] EWCA Civ 1746, the Court of Appeal considered two main issues relating to the scope of the Data Protection Act 1998: the meaning of 'personal data' and whether manual records could be said to have been held in 'a relevant filing system' for the purposes of the Act. The Court came to the conclusion that 'a relevant filing system' is limited to one in which the files are structured or referenced in such a way as clearly to indicate at the outset of the search whether specific information capable of amounting to personal data on an individual requesting it is held within the system and, if so, in which file or files it is held; and that has, as part of its own structure or referencing mechanism, a sufficiently sophisticated and detailed means of readily indicating whether and where in an individual file or files specific criteria or information about the applicant can be easily located.

The Public Interest Disclosure Act 1998

The Act (PIDA) came into force on 2 July 1999 and introduced employment protection rights for workers in most employments who are obliged to disclose information in the public interest. The legislation is often referred to as the 'whistle-blowing' law. The protection applies, however, only to so-called protected disclosures where there is a reasonable belief of wrongdoing in one of the following categories:

- A criminal offence has been committed or is likely to be committed.
- A person has failed, is failing or is likely to fail to comply with any legal obligation to which he is subject.
- A miscarriage of justice has occurred or is likely to occur.
- The health or safety of any individual has been, is being or is likely to be endangered.
- The environment has been, is being or is likely to be damaged.
- That information tending to show any matters falling within any one of the preceding paragraphs has been, is being or is likely to be deliberately concealed.

Certain posts in national security and law and order employments are excluded from the Act's provisions: the Security Service, the Secret Intelligence Service, staff at Government Communications Headquarters and police officers.

The Act defines how workers must disclose information if they are to be afforded legal protection: to their employer; to a legal adviser in order to obtain advice; to a Minister of the Crown where certain types of state employers or public bodies are concerned; to a person appointed by government; or to persons other than those in any of the preceding categories subject to certain conditions, which include the disclosure being made in good faith, based on reasonable grounds of belief and not for financial gain.

Occupational health workers in particular, as well as human resource specialists and general managers, can have access to information that could be covered by the Act. Any proposed disclosure, or 'blowing of a whistle', could result in disciplinary action or even criminal allegations, so it would be sensible to seek advice from a professional body and lawyers before any disclosure is made. This applies even where there is pressure from work colleagues or trade unions to make the disclosure, bearing in mind the competing ethics of disclosure and confidentiality.

The essential feature of a protected disclosure or whistle-blowing case is that the disclosures inherent in the procedure must have been made in good faith. The reasonable belief of the whistle-blower is more important than whether the matter of concern is true or arises from any actual wrongdoing. The employment tribunals will establish the facts and weigh up what may be the malice of a disaffected employee against the disingenuous explanation of an employer. An

---

Case law

There is a growing casebook on PIDA cases, which are often complex and highly specific to particular circumstances and individual facts. It is wise to take proper advice should an employee feel that they need to make a protected disclosure.

The Employment Tribunal supported the correct refusal taken by an occupational health nurse who refused to divulge health records of an individual. In *Cooke* v. *West Yorkshire Probation Board* (2004) ET 1800941/2004, Ms Cooke refused the HR manager's demand to see the health screening form of a person who had recovered from hepatitis and had been passed fit for work. Human resources nevertheless took the file and read the confidential medical information. Ms Cooke complained about this and eventually claimed constructive dismissal. The tribunal found that the principal reason for dismissal was unfair in that the real reason was because Ms Cooke had made a protected disclosure.

The following cases were reported by IDS Brief in a feature article on whistle-blowing.[4]

In *Dudin* v. *Salisbury District Council* ET Case No. 3102263/03, Dudin made a disclosure about bullying and harassment in the workplace to the Council's Scrutiny Panel, which was responsible for reviewing decisions made and actions taken by the Council. Since the matter related to the health and safety of individuals at work, and the HSE is

Cont.

the enforcing authority for district councils, the HSE, not the Scrutiny Panel, was the appropriate 'person' for disclosure under s. 43F. Dudin's disclosure was not protected because it was not made in the prescribed manner.

In *Herron* v. *Wintercomfort for the Homeless* (2003) ET Case No. 1502519/03, Herron was a supported housing project worker who gave information to the police about a former client who had died, apparently as a result of domestic violence. In the tribunal's view, the qualifying disclosure warranted protection under the Act as the relevant failure was that a murder had apparently been committed. The tribunal also gave weight to the fact that disclosure was made to the police, as this was relevant to the issue of reasonableness under the legislation.

Street v. *Derbyshire Unemployed Workers' Centre* [2004] IRLR 687 is a case that illustrates the need for good faith and reasonable belief when protected disclosures are made. Ms Street was employed as an administrator at Derbyshire Unemployed Workers' Centre (DUWC), which was funded by various bodies including Chesterfield Borough Council (CBC). DUWC was managed by a non-employed, elected committee. Ms Street wrote to CBC's treasurer making various complaints about the centre's employed coordinator. She later showed a copy of her letter to a member of DUWC's management committee. The coordinator's conduct was investigated and he was exonerated. DUWC then carried out disciplinary proceedings against Ms Street, which resulted in her dismissal for gross misconduct and breach of trust. Ms Street brought proceedings in the Employment Tribunal claiming automatically unfair dismissal for having made protected disclosures. The tribunal held that the complaints she had made were qualifying disclosures that showed she reasonably believed that her colleague had failed to comply with legal obligations contained in his contract of employment. However, they considered that the disclosures were not protected because they had been made not in good faith but on the basis of her personal antagonism towards him. She therefore lost her case on that ground, even though she had passed some of the other tests required by the Act. The case then went to the Employment Appeals Tribunal. They considered that in deciding whether an applicant acts in good faith, the tribunal has to assess the motive for his or her making allegations. The decision of the Employment Tribunal was therefore upheld. The case moved on to the Court of Appeal, which subsequently upheld the EAT decision. A disclosure cannot be made in good faith if an ulterior motive of malice was the main purpose for making it. The purpose of the Public Interest Disclosure Act is not to promote the ability of people to resolve personal grudges but to protect those who make disclosures in the public interest.

In the case of *Lingard* v. *HM Prison Service* (2004) ET Case No. 1802862/04, the Leeds employment tribunal awarded £477,000 to an employee who was unfairly dismissed for having made a protected disclosure. The employee claimed that she had been badly treated as a result of having reported incidents of prisoners being bullied. The tribunal hearing the case earlier upheld her claim for unfair constructive dismissal on the ground of a protected disclosure. The tribunal judgment on the remedy awarded a basic award of £3915; a compensatory award of £470,687.90 in respect of future loss of earnings and loss of pension rights; and a further £3000 in respect of injury to feelings. At the liability hearing, the tribunal found that the employer had made a deliberate decision to reveal the employee's name as the whistle-blower, and had thereafter failed to protect her from the consequences of the disclosure of her name. In the tribunal's view, the employer totally failed to accept that the employee was genuine and honest in her disclosures and was seriously at risk as a result of making them, principally because it did not wish to face up to the unpleasant truths that were emerging. The size of the award may bring employers to focus anew on the consequences of failing properly to manage whistle-blowing claims at work.

effective whistle-blowing policy will ensure that the employer communicates the fact that complaints will be taken seriously and that no detriment will result from any complaint or grievance so raised.

The Human Rights Act 1998

The Act came into operation in October 2000, the basis of the legislation being to ensure that United Kingdom law is in compliance with the European Convention on Human Rights. There are responsibilities for public authorities, including the professional bodies, to undertake duties formerly imposed on the government. The Act incorporates the rights established by the European Convention on Human Rights. These are:

(1) The right to life.
(2) Prohibition of torture and inhuman or degrading punishment.
(3) Prohibition of slavery or compulsory labour.
(4) Liberty and security of the person.
(5) Fair and public trial without undue delay.
(6) Freedom from retrospective criminal law.
(7) No punishment without legislation.
(8) Respect for privacy in family life, home and correspondence, freedom of thought, conscience and religion.
(9) Freedom of expression.
(10) Freedom of assembly and association.
(11) Marriage and family.
(12) Prohibition of discrimination.
(13) Peaceful enjoyment of property and possessions.
(14) Education.
(15) Free elections.
(16) Not to be subjected to the death penalty.

The Human Rights Act provides that it is unlawful for public authorities such as courts and tribunals, local authorities and health trusts to breach any article of the Convention.

The occupational health profession has interests that cover medical and employment matters in which there is a continuing conflict between the employee/patient/client's right to confidentiality, and the employer's need to know whether a person is fit for work and why any fitness might be qualified to some degree. Confidentiality in the work place includes a human rights perspective along with the individual's right to private and family life because – as provided in Article 8, for example – improper release of medical records could constitute a breach of human rights. The principal area of concern with regard to records and reports is in respect of this privacy right of the individual, overlapping with the provisions of the Data Protection Act 1998 and general ethical considerations. Among these are the use of covert investigations and transmission of information about individuals to third parties including employers (see also Regulation of Investigatory Powers Act 2000).

Occupational health perspectives

The duty of confidentiality

One of the most difficult aspects of occupational health practice arises when occupational health nurses and doctors are asked to divulge information about an employee's health by an employer who is concerned about that employee's absences record or ability to do his job. Practitioners say that they are often asked to divulge information about employees' health that is confidential medical information. Advice on confidentiality is the most requested topic by members of the Royal College of Nursing says Carol Bannister, the RCN's National Adviser on occupational health. There is anecdotal evidence from feedback on concerns expressed by nurses that occupational health staff stress arises from the conflict with management over this very topic. Often, it would seem, this is because there is a misunderstanding of what the employer wants and needs to know, what information the employee wants to release, and what the occupational health practitioner thinks the employer needs to know.

It is a requirement that the employee, in choosing to give or withhold consent, does so as an informed party. He must know, for example, what if any medical records are being disclosed with a medical report.[5] We repeat that each case will turn on its own facts and circumstances. Sometimes it will be helpful if an employer can be told of an employee's medical condition: for example, if someone is diabetic and needs an adjustment to breaks and meal times for medication and management of his condition. Provided the employee agrees to this, the information can be reported. Sometimes only a prognosis may be relevant and/or able to be given. The overriding issues for occupational health professionals include ensuring that they and the employee understand the possible implications of withholding information: an employer is expected to make decisions based on what he knows or ought reasonably to know, so not giving the relevant facts could in some circumstances not be in the employee's best interests. On the other hand, some medical conditions are simply not relevant to the report and could even mislead a non-clinical person if revealed. These are not easy issues.

The overriding issues are consent and confidentiality. At the very worst, occupational health professionals can be sued, disciplined and dismissed by an employer, as well as struck off by their professional body for breaches of confidentiality. The health professionals are obliged to follow the law on privacy and confidentiality and they are expected to follow their relevant codes of ethics and professional conduct standards.[6,7] There is a legal and ethical duty of confidence on the part of the health professionals in their relationship with the client or patient. Therefore the issue of keeping records and writing reports is a complex one and is often seen by the occupational health practitioners as fraught with the danger of breaching confidentiality. Where there is uncertainty, there is a tendency to err on the side of caution. There is a benefit to this caution in that the discretion of the occupational health professions does tend to engender trust in those who confide in them.

For occupational health nurses, one of the basic requirements for practice is that they should be competent to manage inappropriate requests to disclose personal health information without informed consent of individuals. Another essential obligation is to manage the safe storage and retrieval of occupational health records.[8] The expert practitioner should be providing leadership and managing the conflict relating to confidentiality of data collection, recording, retrieval and dissemination.

Occupational health physicians' ethical guidance is under review at the time of writing, but existing guidance from the Faculty of Occupational Medicine[9] includes the confidentiality aspects of practice and states quite clearly that 'the individual occupational health record is a confidential medical record to which the principles of medical confidentiality apply'. It goes on to say that both the occupational health physician and occupational health nurse are, jointly or separately, responsible for all clinical information and its storage in whatever format. This will of course depend on whether there is both an occupational health nurse and doctor employed by the company and so allows for those situations where only one discipline is present or employed. Such 'individual occupational health records' are one form of a health record mentioned earlier in this chapter and as such are regarded as sensitive data under the DPA.

For both doctors and nurses, proper record keeping is regarded as an integral part of patient or client care. The Nursing and Midwifery Council regard it as a fundamental part of practice[10] and as a tool for professional practice, saying that 'it is not an optional extra to be fitted in if circumstances allow'. The General Medical Council requires that doctors keep clear, accurate, legible and contemporaneous records.[11]

There are several factors that contribute to effective record keeping. From the list in Fig. 2.1 it can be seen that there are a number of points to be considered in occupational health practice as these records may be required at a later date for legal reasons such as employment tribunals or personal injury claims against the employer. Also, the patient/client has access rights to his or her individual records, so they should be written in such a way that they can be understood, and can be seen by a third party if the patient/client gives written permission. It follows that the records should be relevant, should comply with proper standards and be comprehensible to the individual. Dimond[12] recommends that when photocopies are made of records the individual's name, details and date should be on each side of the paper to avoid confusion when single-sided photocopies are taken. This will prevent them from being lost when there is a risk of separation. The NMC suggests that all alterations are dated, timed and signed to avoid confusion

Clinical audit

If keeping patient and client records is an integral part of patient/client care then the process should be audited, because audit forms an essential part of clinical governance. Clinical governance is a framework that helps all clinicians to improve quality continuously and safeguard standards of patient/client care[13] and includes:

Records should:
- Be factual, consistent and accurate.
- Be written as soon as possible after the event has occurred, providing current information on the care and condition of the patient or client.
- Be written clearly and in such a manner that the text cannot be erased.
- Be written in such a manner that any alterations or additions are dated, timed and signed in such a way that the original entry can still be read clearly.
- Be accurately dated, timed and signed with the signature printed alongside the first entry.
- Not include abbreviations, jargon, meaningless phrases, irrelevant speculation and offensive subjective statements.
- Be readable on old photocopies.
- Be written with the involvement of the patient, client or carer.
- Be written in terms that the patient/client can understand.
- Be consecutive.
- Identify problems that have arisen and the action taken to rectify them.
- Provide clear evidence of the care planned, the decisions made, the care delivered and the information shared.

Fig. 2.1 Factors that contribute to effective record keeping (Nursing and Midwifery Council 2005).

- clinical audit
- risk management
- evidence-based practice
- customer input and feedback
- clinical supervision
- continuing professional development

Clinical audit is a method of judging the way one works against evidence-based good practice. It can be used to look at specific activities in occupational health or as a self audit on such things as record keeping by peer review.[14] Agius describes clinical audit as involving a process of repeating cycles, which should result in a progressive improvement and eventually lead to sustained assurance of quality in particular areas, while identifying needs and methods of audit in new areas.[15] This concept has been termed the 'audit cycle' (see Fig. 2.2).

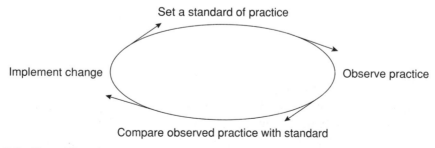

Fig. 2.2 The audit cycle.

By auditing record-keeping procedures, assessment can be made of the standard of the records and areas identified for improvement. Indeed, Part 4 of the Data Protection Act Code of Practice suggests that an impact assessment of sensitive data is carried out and says that this involves:

- Identifying clearly the purposes for which health information is to be collected and the benefits this is likely to deliver.
- Identifying any likely adverse impact of collecting and holding the information.
- Considering alternatives to collecting and holding such information.
- Taking into account the obligations that arise from collecting and holding health information.
- Judging whether collecting and holding health information is justified.

Therefore, when undertaking a clinical audit for record keeping in occupational health practice it is essential to consider the DPA's Code of Practice and the advice on impact assessment.

The Code goes on to suggest actions that may have an adverse impact on keeping health information or records, such as the access to electronic files by IT department workers, so care must be taken when setting up electronic health record systems to ensure that there is access only to those who have a legitimate business to know. The Code also outlines some of the ethical issues discussed in Chapter 3 about health surveillance and the justification for keeping health records, as well as the need for risk assessment, health surveillance requirements and the keeping of health information. All of these factors indicate the importance and necessity for occupational health practitioners to identify for themselves questions such as: What is an individual occupational health record? What are the COSHH and health records retention requirements? What does the DPA Code suggest as guidance, and how does this relate to justified business needs? Where do professional and legal confidentiality rules apply? Does the employee give consent to disclosures? What is health information to which the employer may have access, such as the results of health surveillance? Undertaking an impact assessment and clinical audit will help to answer these questions and clarify the issues to ensure best practice.

Writing reports

Occupational health professionals are required to write a number of reports to management on a variety of occupational health and health and safety topics. These include reports on:

- Pre-employment fitness to work of an individual.
- Health surveillance test results.
- Management referrals to determine fitness to work following accident or illness.
- Environmental or workstation assessments.
- The business case for new equipment, staff, resources or health promotion activities.

These are important documents. Some reports will be instigated by the occupational health service, such as those making a business case, while others will be in response to a request from management. For occupational health practice it is best that management referrals to occupational health are made in writing, clearly stating what management wants to know. A sample template management referral form is given at Appendix 4.

The most important aspect of the report is what is its purpose and what is required: in other words what to include, what to leave out, and who is it for? In the practical world of business a report conveys information and usually has recommendations from the person who has investigated the subject in detail. Whatever the report, it is important to look at the question being asked and the purpose for the request. This clarity and confidence can help to avoid tension in the relationship between management and occupational health.

Effective communication is a two-way process. A useful and valid report will not benefit the individual or the employer in a referral – for example, to advise on the fitness of someone to undertake a job – when the information in the referral request is vague or incomplete. Further information and clarification should be sought in these circumstances. Pre-employment health assessment is an instance where the stakeholders all have different interests. Whitaker's research on pre-employment health assessment has shown that there are a variety of problems in practice and that many health assessment forms may be asking unnecessary and intrusive questions.[16]

It is stressed that there is a need for clear policies for both management and occupational health, particularly in areas such as pre-employment, sickness absence, alcohol and drug-testing referrals. The policies should outline clear guidance for all concerned. Management needs more than just brief statements saying that someone is 'unfit for work'. What they need to know or have some idea about is a prognosis and – where appropriate and helpful to the employee and employer – a diagnosis, an indication of how long the employee may be expected to be off sick and whether any adjustments to the workplace or job are indicated (this is dealt with in more detail in later chapters).

This means that proper report-writing skills should be developed. It is helpful for reports to follow a standard format encompassing relevant information, to include:

- *An introduction:* stating the topic in question; who asked for the report and why; the background; how the information required has been obtained.
- *Findings and discussion:* what the findings are and their implications. Where this is a report on an individual employee's health it must be remembered that confidential medical information cannot be given without the employee's written consent.
- *Summary, conclusion and recommendations:* a sentence or paragraph to sum up and draw a conclusion, which is then followed by recommendations such as workplace or working duty adjustments.
- *Date and signature.*

More details on report writing are available from The Plain English Campaign at www.plainenglish.co.uk/reportguide.html.

Record keeping and report writing are fundamental aspects of occupational health practice. Not only do they help to protect patients, clients and the practitioner but they also serve to demonstrate high standards of practice to others.

References

1. Public Health (Control of Disease) Act 1984 and Public Health (Infectious Diseases) Regulations 1988 SI No. 1546.
2. Kloss, Diana (2005) Medical records and confidentiality. In: *Occupational Health Law*, 4th edn. Blackwell Publishing, Oxford.
3. Health and Safety Executive (1999) *Health Surveillance at Work*. HSE, London.
4. Incomes Data Services (2005) Whistle-blowing update (feature article). *IDS Brief* 794.
5. Kloss, Diana (2005) *Occupational Health Law*, 4th edn. Blackwell Publishing, Oxford.
6. Nursing and Midwifery Council (2004) *The NMC Code of Professional Conduct: Standards for Conduct, Performance and Ethics*. NMC, London.
7. General Medical Council (2001) *Standards for Practice*. GMC, London.
8. Royal College of Nursing (2005) *Competencies: An Integrated Career and Competency Framework for Occupational Health Nursing*. NMC, London.
9. Faculty of Occupational Medicine (1999) *Guidance on Ethics for Occupational Physicians*. Faculty of Occupational Medicine, London.
10. Nursing and Midwifery Council (2005) *Guidelines for Records and Record Keeping*. NMC, London.
11. General Medical Council (2001) *Standards for Practice*. GMC, London.
12. Dimond, B. (2005) Exploring the principles of good record keeping in nursing. *British Journal of Nursing*, **14** (8), 460–62.
13. Royal College of Nursing (2003) *Clinical Governance: An RCN Resource Guide*. RCN, London.
14. Royal College of Nursing (1999) *Occupational Health Audit: A Guide for Occupational Health Nurses*. RCN, London.
15. www.agius.com.hew/audit/1.htm
16. Whitaker, S. & Aw, T. C. (1995) Audit of pre-employment assessment by occupational health departments. *NHS Journal of Occupational Medicine*, **45** (2), 75–80.

Chapter 3
Health Surveillance

According to government statistics, 40 million working days were lost as a result of work-related illness in 2001–2002.[1] Yet work-related illness can be prevented and absenteeism can be controlled. Health and safety legislation exists to prevent ill health arising from the workplace. The Health and Safety Executive supports employers by producing guidelines and codes of practice on health and safety legislation and specific regulations. These codes and guides help employers to understand what is required to provide a safe and healthy workplace. One of the most specific aspects of ill health prevention or reduction that requires explanation is health surveillance. The Health and Safety Executive states:

> 'Health surveillance is about putting in place systematic, regular and appropriate procedures to detect early signs of work-related ill health among employees exposed to certain health risks; and acting on the results.'[2]

The HSE notes that the primary benefit of health surveillance is to detect any adverse health effects at an early stage. This will enable medical conditions to be detected early so that treatment may commence and the health effects be reduced or minimised. Therefore it can be said that health surveillance alone does not control or prevent occupational ill health; it is but one element of an integrated control programme, which includes a hierarchy of control measures according to the type of hazard and the exposure.

Legal perspectives

There is a statutory requirement on employers to safeguard, so far as is reasonably practicable, the health and safety of everyone on their premises. The obligations extend to ensuring the health and safety of all employees, other workers on site and the public. They also extend to placing health and safety responsibilities upon every individual at work.

Failure to comply with the prescribed legal standards can result in criminal prosecution and civil action claims. In addition to general civil remedies for damages for injuries suffered in the workplace, the law provides for punishment through prosecutions under the Health and Safety at Work etc. Act 1974 (HASWA) and subordinate legislation such as the Management of Health and Safety at Work Regulations 1999 (MHSWR) SI No. 3242, the Control of Substances Hazardous to Health Regulations 2002 SI No. 2677 (as amended) (COSHH) and a wealth of further legislation and supporting regulations.

HASWA sets out general duties applicable to workplaces and all workers and persons in the work premises. It gives powers of enforcement to the officers of the Health and Safety Executive, which itself is responsible to the Health and Safety Commission, and imposes duties on the entire spectrum of workers – the self-employed, sub-contractors and workers at every level. It also protects visitors on the premises. HASWA marked a turning point in health and safety law, providing for prevention (through improvement notices and prohibition notices) in addition to the threat of criminal punishment for contravention of its provisions. It is the cornerstone of modern health and safety law. The Factories Act 1961 and the Offices, Shops and Railway Premises Act 1963 are now largely repealed, except for their useful definitions of types of workplace.

HASWA places duties on employers, the self-employed, designers, manufacturers and employees. There are also particular responsibilities for the health and safety of certain people such as night workers, pregnant workers and young, inexperienced or trainee workers. Risk assessments that take account of the specific risks that can face young and inexperienced workers and those working while pregnant must be carried out as part of health surveillance. There are also restrictions on the work young people can be employed to do, their working hours and special requirements as to the provision and use of work equipment for young workers. Details can be found on the HSE website: www.hse.gov.uk.

The legal framework is based upon statute law and common law. Statute includes criminal law and is the written law consisting of Acts of Parliament, Regulations and Orders, such as the HASWA. Common law is the system of precedents used by the courts to determine outcomes based on past cases.

What is health surveillance?

Within the legal duties imposed on everyone at work is a requirement to carry out health and safety surveillance as defined by the relevant regulations. Under regulation 6 of MHSWR:

'Every employer shall ensure that his employees are provided with such health surveillance as is appropriate having regard to the risks to their health and safety which are identified by the assessment.'

Carrying out the health surveillance process provides a key determinant in meeting the legal requirements of health and safety responsibilities. It is vital to the duty, practicability and reasonableness tests should a case come to court.

Taking preventative and analytical steps not only ensures compliance with legal obligations, but also can help to prevent work-related ill health. This is achieved by controlling and assessing risk factors through effective health surveillance programmes.

Confusion often arises from the difficulty in ascertaining which aspects of health surveillance are mandatory legal duties and which are good practice but have no direct legal obligation ascribed to them. In stating the latter, employers need to bear in mind their general responsibilities under the Health and Safety at Work Act 1974 'to ensure so far as is reasonably practicable, the health, safety and welfare of all employees' and they need to have evidence of their good practice to show that they have made efforts to comply with this duty.

The MHSWR 1999 and the COSHH Regulations 2002 set out the main areas of work that require, as a legal duty, health surveillance to be carried out. These include, but are not limited to, the following example categories:

- Suitable and sufficient assessment of risks to health and safety in the workplace (for all employees) and on the premises (for other persons on site).
- Pre-placement and then annual medical examinations to assess fitness for work, under any specific rules or requirements such as the Ionising Radiations Regulations 1999 SI No. 3232 and the Diving at Work Regulations 1997 SI No. 2776
- Any initial medical examination and subsequent annual or bi-annual medical assessments such as those for pilots and air traffic controllers as required by relevant legislation promulgated by the responsible regulatory body.[3]
- Any obligatory eyesight and medical checks as required for certain jobs such as HGV or PSV drivers or crane operators within dock premises.[4]
- Compliance with the provisions of regulations concerned with any specified and particular function such as the Health and Safety (Display Screen Equipment) Regulations 1992 SI No. 2792 (as amended 2002), Manual Handling Operations Regulations 1992 SI No. 2793 (as amended 2002), Personal Protective Equipment at Work Regulations 1992 SI No. 2966 (as amended 2002 SI No. 1144) and Control of Noise at Work Regulations 2005 SI No. 1643.
- Fitness for work health assessments, which must be offered to night workers under the Working Time Regulations 1998 SI No. 1833.
- Where chemical and biological agents are present in the workplace, health surveillance may be required under the Control of Substances Hazardous to Health Regulations 2002 SI No. 2677 (COSHH).
- Where exposure to particular hazards or materials is a factor, compliance with medical examinations must be carried out as required: for example, exposure to asbestos, lead, compressed air.

The above list is illustrative and not exhaustive. Further advice must be sought from the controlling authorities and needs to be updated on a regular basis. The HSE is an excellent starting point. There is an Approved Code of Practice, which provides an excellent guide to health surveillance. Other authorities offer helpful guidance as to vocational requirements for the professions they regulate, such as the Civil Aviation Authority for pilots, air traffic controllers and aircrew.

The Employment Medical Advisory Service (EMAS) conducts medical examinations through its Appointed Doctors (ADs) who work under the supervision of HSE occupational health specialist physicians. It is one of the roles of EMAS to carry out examinations of workers and assess fitness to work as required to comply with statutory health surveillance requirements.[5]

Manufacturers of machinery and equipment also provide essential information as to how their products should be used and of dangers or hazards to be avoided.

It is worth noting that practices and advice about machinery usage does change from time to time. Notification can come from a manufacturer's or supplier's update letter, or through current information provided with newly purchased equipment, or through trade journal or newspaper notices. Any such changes should be tracked, noted and communicated to the workforce.

The HSE provides essential guidance under its Approved Codes of Practice for a full range of potentially hazardous work situations. The HASWA, MHSWR and COSHH all impose certain statutory duties generally and which, under HASWA, extend to risks arising from work activities, i.e. risks to employees and other persons. The MHSWR provides a broad framework for controlling health and safety at work. COSHH provides a framework aimed at controlling the risks from hazardous substances including infectious agents.

Under HASWA, employers are in general required to:

- Assess the risks in their workplace.
- Use competent help to apply health and safety legislation.
- Establish procedures to use if an employee is presented with serious and imminent danger.
- Cooperate and coordinate health and safety if there is more than one employer in a workplace.

Under COSHH, employers are required to:

- Assess the risks of exposure to hazardous substances in their workplace.
- Prevent exposure, or substitute with a less hazardous substance or process/ method if possible.
- Control exposure to hazards if prevention or substitution is not reasonably practicable.
- Maintain, examine and test any control measures.
- Provide information, instruction and training for employees.
- Provide health surveillance of employees if appropriate.

Health and safety policy

Section 2 (3) of HASWA imposes a duty on every employer of five or more persons to prepare, and bring to the notice of their employees, a written statement of their general policy with respect to the health and safety at work of employees.

Health and safety policy statements usually consist of three parts:

- A statement of intent, which is a declaration of the employer's commitment to providing a safe and healthy workplace and environment. This will also cover essentials, with the object of ensuring, so far as is reasonably practicable, the health and safety at work of every employee: for example, the arrangements for ensuring the safe use, handling, storage and transport of 'articles and substances' that are inherently or potentially dangerous; the provision of comprehensive information, instruction, training and supervision; the maintenance of the workplace in a safe and risk-free condition, the provision

of safe means of access to and egress from the workplace; and the provision and maintenance of a safe and healthy working environment with adequate welfare facilities and arrangements.
- Details of responsibilities for health and safety throughout the organisation.
- Details of safe systems of work/safe working practices for all work activities. Safety problems and hazards vary from industry to industry, from employer to employer and from site to site. Policies should be tailored to the employer's undertaking and reflect the known issues highlighted through the health surveillance programmes.

The policy will take account of the workplace and working practice requirements and set out clear objectives to preserve and protect the health, safety and welfare at work of each of the employees, including persons not directly within their employment.

HASWA also states that the policy statement must be reviewed as appropriate, e.g. on the introduction of new processes, activities or machinery. This is a crucial part of the health surveillance function. Good reporting, recommendations, action plans and reviews are essential.

Legal redress: criminal cases

Criminal prosecutions can be brought by individuals but this is still not common in health and safety matters. The Health and Safety Executive and local authorities have responsibility for enforcing the criminal law where breaches of health and safety rules are alleged. In those cases where deaths are involved, parties may be prosecuted by the Crown Prosecution Service.

The Corporate Manslaughter Bill looks set to introduce the possibility of this additional criminal charge. The new law, which is in the process of coming into effect, will create the specific offence of corporate manslaughter in which an organisation will be guilty of corporate manslaughter if its senior managers arrange for its activities to be carried out in such a way as to cause a person's death through the gross breach of a duty of care owed to that person. Punishment on conviction will be an unlimited fine. Instead of named scapegoats being sought, the actual organisation will be liable. A responsible individual could also be charged separately, however, if he is alleged to have caused death, with concurrent charges still able to be brought against that individual.

Senior management will be closely involved in any prosecution since the company or organisation will be the corporate body carrying responsibility for their acts or omissions. A person will be defined as a senior manager if he has significant responsibility for 'the making of decisions about how the whole or a substantial part of its activities are to be managed or organised, or the actual managing or organising of the whole or a substantial part of those activities'.[6]

The affected individual in a criminal case generally has the status of victim/ witness and has no control over the running of the criminal case or its outcome. Civil cases are brought independently and may be funded privately by insurance,

Case law

The train derailment near Hatfield on 17 October 2000 led to the loss of four lives, with 70 people injured. The investigation into the derailment was undertaken jointly by HSE and the British Transport Police, with the latter in the lead.

On 9 July 2003 the Crown Prosecution Service (CPS) announced that six individuals had been charged with the manslaughter of the four people who died in the Hatfield derailment and with breaches of provisions under the Health and Safety at Work etc Act 1974 (HASWA). A further six individuals had been served with summonses for breaches of HASWA. In addition, summonses for manslaughter and breaches of HASWA were served on Network Rail (formerly Railtrack plc) as the infrastructure controller and Balfour Beatty Rail Infrastructure Services Ltd (formerly Balfour Beatty Rail Maintenance Ltd) as the maintenance contractor.

At a hearing on 1 September 2004, the manslaughter charges against Railtrack, and manslaughter and health and safety charges against some of these individuals (employed by Railtrack), were dismissed. On 14 July 2005, the Old Bailey Judge dismissed manslaughter charges against five executives – three from Railtrack and two from Balfour Beatty – accused of the manslaughter of the four people who died in the Hatfield derailment. A corporate manslaughter charge against engineering firm Balfour Beatty was also dismissed by the Judge. On 18 July 2005, Balfour Beatty pleaded guilty to a health and safety charge relating to the derailment.

On Tuesday 6 September 2005, Network Rail (Railtrack) was found guilty of health and safety charges, and the five individuals tried were found not guilty. On 3 October 2005, the CPS offered no evidence on health and safety charges against four individuals, and these were dismissed. On 7 October 2005, Balfour Beatty was fined £10 million and Network Rail (Railtrack) was fined £3.5 million; they were also ordered to pay £300,000 each in prosecution costs.[7]

through union membership cover, or on a conditional fee arrangement (sometimes referred to as a 'no win, no fee' arrangement).

Criminal cases are heard in the magistrates' courts where the powers of sentencing are limited to fines as set out under HASWA and supporting regulations. It is important to note that Employer Liability Insurance schemes do not cover payment of fines made by the courts. Magistrates may fine and sentence up to defined levels and limited terms of imprisonment. The Crown Court has unlimited powers of fines and can impose higher prison sentences. Criminal courts can award compensation payments to victims of accidents but the amounts paid out tend not to be commensurate with the suffering caused to the injured person. The same limitations apply to payments made under the Criminal Injuries Compensation Authority scheme. As a result there will often be a civil court action conducted by the individual following a criminal action, in order to pursue financial recompense through a damages claim.

As noted previously, the legal framework is enacted through statute and common law. In respect of statutory health and safety matters, this is achieved through:

- Acts (Employers' Liability (Compulsory Insurance) Act 1969, Employers' Liability (Defective Equipment) Act 1969)

- Regulations
- approved codes of practice
- guidance notes

The HSE (Health and Safety Executive) is the principal appointed body for ensuring adequate arrangements for the enforcement of statutory provisions. Inspectors have extensive powers:

- To enter premises.
- To be accompanied by police if necessary.
- To bring assistants or materials or equipment with them.
- To examine and investigate.
- To direct that the premises, or part of them, or anything there, be left as they are for the purpose of examination or investigation.
- To take measurements, photographs or recordings as necessary.
- To take samples of substances and of the atmosphere.
- To require any article or substances for dismantling, testing or possession as necessary for examination or evidence. This includes the power to inspect and copy books, documents, etc.

If an inspector considers that there is contravention of the regulations, or a failure to comply with statutory provisions, then he can serve an improvement notice. This will specify the reason for the notice and a specified time limit within which rectification must take place – usually not less than 21 days. Improvement notices can be served on anyone – manager, employee, supplier of equipment. The main purpose of the improvement notice is to require those upon whom it is served to do whatever is necessary or to cease to do whatever the notice identifies as a contravention. During this time the person's liability for criminal or civil liability remains extant.

If the inspector considers that there is a risk of serious personal injury, then a prohibition notice may be served on the person or company. Prohibition notices have to include:

- The statement of the inspector that in his opinion there is a risk of serious personal injury.
- The matters that give rise to this opinion.
- The relevant statutory provisions that give rise to the reasons for his opinion
- The direction to cease the activities noted.

There is a right of appeal against improvement or prohibition notices. It must be exercised within the specified time limit. An appeal against an improvement notice has the effect of suspending its operation pending the hearing of the appeal. A prohibition notice takes immediate effect, unless a tribunal expressly lifts the notice pending the outcome of the appeal.

As well as serving an improvement or prohibition notice, an inspector can prosecute anyone who has allegedly contravened a statutory provision, or who has allegedly failed to discharge a duty to which he is subject, or who falsifies documents, or who fails to comply with an improvement or prohibition notice.

Legal redress: civil cases

The burden of proof in criminal cases is greater than that required in civil law. In criminal cases the burden of proof is upon the prosecution to establish that the case against the accused is 'sure', or what is known as 'beyond reasonable doubt'. In civil cases the burden of proof hinges upon the concept of a reasonable belief based upon the balance of probabilities. It is therefore perfectly possible, as evidenced in case law, for there to be a different outcome of two matters related to the one case, when tested at criminal and at civil law.

The key requirements that will be tested against the employer's compliance with the duty of care are:

- Providing a safe place of work.
- Providing a safe means of access to and egress from the place of work.
- Providing a safe system of work.
- Providing adequate equipment and materials.
- Employing competent fellow employees.
- Protecting employees from unnecessary risk of injury.

All of these factors relate to the 'safe system of work' (HASWA section 2 (2) a and c), which includes such matters as manning of operations, equipment and supervision.

Key points to note in developing safe systems of work will include:

- Consideration of any single issue that might impeach upon the safety of the whole safe system of work, e.g. in quarry blasting, is the warning time sufficient?
- Operations so inherently dangerous as to not be performed at all.
- Consultation with staff.
- Compliance with statutory requirements.

The duty to provide a safe system of work is not an absolute one. The duty is to take reasonable steps to provide a system that will be reasonably safe, having regard to the dangers necessarily inherent in the operation. While evidence of established practice is valid, the courts will also look at current best practice.

The extent of the duty will take account of:

- The extent of the danger.
- The likelihood of accident occurrence.
- The steps needed to eliminate all risks and the cost of doing so.

Employers are under a duty to take reasonable care to ensure the safety of their employees. That duty extends to ensuring that employees are not subjected to unnecessary risk of injury.

Where a risk is not reasonably foreseeable, the employee's claim will succeed only if he can show that current industry knowledge in the relevant work at the relevant time was such that the employer knew or ought to have known of that risk.

Note should also be taken of the following matters relating to causal work factors and reasonable care:

*   Mental and physical health risk.
*   Industrial disease and injury: causal factors.

Case law

The famous case of *Stokes* v. *GKN (Nuts and Bolts) Ltd* [1968] 1 WLR 1776 confirms the legal duty based on the test of what an employer knew or ought to have known. In this case it was held that the company physician did not tell employees that they were at risk of scrotal cancer by wearing overalls that were steeped in mineral oils. Nor did he tell the employer. The court held that the company ought to have known of the risk even though the doctor had withheld the information. Although this case was heard prior to the enactment of HASWA, the courts were even then concerned with the employer's liability for maintaining a safe place and safe system of work. It is today one of the leading case law standards. It leads us to another key factor in health and safety related cases: that of contributory negligence on the part of the employee. In the Stokes case, for example, had the employees known of the risk and continued to wear the contaminated overalls or, in any other situation, carried out a comparably dangerous activity, any damages awarded might have been reduced by reason of contributory negligence.

In another landmark case, *Lane* v. *Shire Roofing Co* [1995] IRLR 493, the concept of contributory negligence was tested in court. Mr Lane was an independent contractor who was doing roofing work when he fell from a ladder and suffered serious head injuries. His damages were cut by 50% because using his own equipment (an unsuitable ladder) in a dangerous way was attributable to the accident in which he fell and injured his back.

Claims for personal injury must be lodged with the court within three years of the cause of action arising. The Limitation Act 1980 allows that general principle to be extended so that actions may also be lodged within three years of the date of knowledge that there is an injury or disease that is attributable to a workplace factor. This was an issue in the asbestos-related claims and the coal miners' claims in which the date of knowledge was accepted by the courts as being later than three years following the injury or disease onset. This is a very important factor to be considered by employers in deciding on the time guidelines they choose to follow in keeping their records of health surveillance under Data Protection compliance standards.

Before court action, the employee can communicate with the employer on the subject of settlement compensation, in order to avoid litigation. This is usually begun on a without prejudice basis and can commence at the start or at any point in the litigation's progress. The possibility that a claim can be settled at an early stage without the need for legal action is a useful consideration. The employee will be wise to take some legal advice as to the potential value of the claim. Unions generally assist their members through all stages of a claim for compensation where there is a reasonable prospect of success. There are many other sources of free or low-cost advice for non-union members, such as the Citizens Advice Bureau, and insurance policies that expressly cover legal expenses or include this as an option: for example, household or car insurance policies.

Special damages are those damages that can be specifically quantified. They are awarded for the actual financial loss sustained, such as:

- Medical expenses.
- Cost of transport to medical appointments such as with a physiotherapist or specialist.
- Expense of relatives visiting the injured person in hospital.
- Value of clothing damaged in the accident.
- Loss of income.
- Expense of domestic and other assistance during recovery.

General damages are notional amounts awarded to compensate for pain, suffering and loss of amenity. General damages are awarded in addition to special damages. The Judicial Studies Board Guidelines set out the general range of damages

Case study: a noise claim[8]

Because it may be many years before the effects of exposure to noise are manifest, the courts are concerned with the difficulties that the claimant has to overcome to make his claim stand. It is not sufficient to say that the noise was deafening between 1960 and 1970, and that is why there is deafness in 2006. The claimant must make clear in the particulars of his claim just what is the nature of his complaint, and must:

- State the dates of exposure to the noise.
- State where the exposure took place.
- Identify the capacity in which the claimant was employed in relation to each workplace of which he complains.
- Identify and describe the duties undertaken at the time of the alleged exposure.
- Provide a sketch plan or diagram of the layout of the workplace identifying the location of each source of noise complained of and showing the proximity of the claimant to the source of noise.
- Identify each source of noise complained of.
- State the frequency of exposure to noise (daily, weekly) and how long each episode lasted.
- Provide expert opinion of the level of noise.
- State the standards or criteria governing safety according to which it is alleged such noise levels were excessive, saying by how much.
- Enumerate complaints made, when and to whom, and for what purpose.
- Describe any available hearing protection, stating when it was made available, where and from whom, and the make and type.
- State when hearing loss and or tinnitus was first noticed.
- State when medical help was sought.
- Describe all other exposure to noise.

to be awarded for injuries, and case law is reported so that lawyers can see how special circumstances affect the value of awards.

Good practice and defences

At civil law, the defence is a question of evidence and the quality of that evidence. Under the criminal law, the nature of the offence must be considered in case there is no defence to be offered. The basic principles of criminal law are set out in HASWA and these are also reflected in the common law duties:

> 'It shall be the duty of every employer to ensure, so far as is reasonably practicable, the health, safety and welfare of all his employees.'

Therefore, defences will centre upon the definitions of:

- duty
- practicability
- reasonableness

These three words form the cornerstones of health surveillance as required by law and by good practice.

An absolute duty requires compliance, regardless of cost: for example, a licence or other legal compliance requirement. There is an implied duty in every contract of employment to safeguard the health and safety of employees.

Practicability covers protection from risk of matters that are feasible, foreseeable and possible.

The word 'reasonable' allows some leeway in terms of balancing the cost of preventative action against the risks involved.

The onus is upon employers to show that it was not practicable to do more than they did to satisfy their duties and requirements, or that there were no more appropriate means practicable than those that they took.

By statute and by the standards of civil law, everyone in the workplace owes a duty of care to everyone else, whatever their status. These general duties include obligations upon every individual to:

- Take reasonable care for their own safety and that of others.
- Cooperate with employer rules and safety standards.
- Not misuse safety devices or other equipment provided.
- Correctly use machinery, substances, equipment, etc.
- Report accidents, hazards or concerns.
- Attend training as required.
- Follow all preventative and protective procedures.
- Comply with emergency procedures.

Contributory negligence on the part of an employee can result in the amount of damages in any civil claim award to them being reduced in proportion to the element to which the employee failed to take reasonable steps to ensure his or her own safety: examples include failing to follow proper procedures; not making use of safety equipment supplied.

Senior employees (supervisors and managers) are responsible for local implementation of rules and legislation, compliance with any requirements of safety inspections and safety committee attendance, and the undertaking of any duties in their job description or any special responsibilities as designated.

Executive or senior management responsibility focuses on the managing director or the most senior executive in an organisation who has overall responsibility for:

- Implementing and monitoring health and safety policy.
- Safe systems of work.
- Safety training.
- Accident investigation.

Management has further responsibilities associated with its supervisory and directing role, and so has a duty to:

- Take top-level responsibility by a named person, with overall duty to oversee policy.
- Monitor and review the policy and its full implementation.
- Ensure safe systems of work.
- Provide training in work systems and health and safety policy development.
- Investigate accidents.
- Establish safety committees, representatives and meetings.
- Comply with safety regulations.
- Ensure health surveillance and risk assessments are undertaken.
- Set standards, and monitor and review for all employees, visitors, contractors, etc.
- Ensure adequate first aid and fire procedures (equipment, inspections, training, alarm tests, etc.).
- Ensure COSHH management and compliance.
- Ensure RIDDOR management and compliance.

These are all elements of the health surveillance duty, and as such will form the basis for good practice and defence against any actions or allegations connected with health and safety at work.

Accident and incident reporting

RIDDOR

The Reporting of Injuries, Diseases and Dangerous Occurrences Regulations 1995 SI No. 3163 (RIDDOR) require designated responsible persons to report to their enforcing authority (generally the Health and Safety Executive or local environmental health department) the following work-related incidents:

- Fatal accidents.
- Major injury accidents/conditions.
- Incidents where, as a result of an accident connected with the workplace, people not at work receive an injury requiring hospital treatment.

- Incidents where a person at work suffers a major injury requiring hospital treatment.
- Accidents causing more than three days' incapacity for work.
- Dangerous occurrences.
- Death of an employee within one year of an injury arising from a notifiable accident or dangerous occurrence.
- Certain work-related diseases.
- Certain matters dealing with the safe supply of gas.

'Accidents' include acts of physical violence suffered at work, or even the threat of such if this was sufficiently alarming as to cause fear of an actual assault. Fatal accidents, major injury accidents/conditions and dangerous occurrences must be reported immediately by the quickest practicable means to the relevant enforcing authority. If there is doubt as to whether the incident is reportable, or as to which authority is the correct one to notify, the advice of the Health and Safety Executive should be obtained. As all employment establishments must by law display the health and safety poster as required by the HSE, which must provide details thereon of the local health and safety office, this would normally be the first point of contact.

Following the initial notification, a written report on the approved form F2508 or F2508A must be sent to the enforcing authority within ten days of the accident or dangerous occurrence. It is now possible to make a report by post, email, telephone or fax via the Incident Contact Centre in Caerphilly:

By post: Incident Contact Centre, Caerphilly Business park, Caerphilly, CF83 3GG
By internet: www.riddor.gov.uk
By telephone: 0845 300 9923
By fax: 0845 300 9924
By email: riddor@natbrit.com

If an employee dies within one year as a result of an accident that is reportable (whether or not it was reported at the time), the employer is required by law to notify the enforcing authority in writing as soon as the death comes to their knowledge.

If the person killed or injured is self-employed or a temporary worker, it is the responsibility of the employer or the person in control of the premises. Therefore if a temporary worker is killed or injured while working on a client's premises, the accident must be reported by the hiring client and, prudently, by the agency also.

In the case of certain specific workplaces (e.g. offshore installations) or types of incident, there are specific regulations that state who is deemed to be 'the responsible person'. For example, in the case of dangerous occurrences arising from transportation by road of dangerous goods, the responsible person will be the holder of the operator's licence or keeper of the vehicle. Road accidents are not in themselves covered by the regulations except where the incident arises from exposure to a substance that is being transported or the loading or unloading of a vehicle, or specified road works, or where a train is involved.

The act of reporting the incident does not confirm liability for the injury or damage but it is a breach of the requirements not to report an incident as required under RIDDOR.

Record keeping and accident books

The responsible person must keep certain records, which must be retained for at least three years from the date on which the entry is made. These include the date and time of the accident or dangerous occurrence, full name and occupation of person affected including nature of the injury, place where the incident occurred and a brief description of the circumstances. Note that under the Data Protection Act 1998 confidentiality rules, the nature of any injury or illness should be retained as sensitive and confidential information.

This information should not be on view in any accident reporting book. The HSE provides a suitable book that provides for meeting this requirement. All employers who normally employ ten or more persons on or about the same premises in connection with a trade or business must keep an accident book[9] at the premises to record all injuries, however minor, for a period of three years from the date of the last entry.

First aid

The general duty of an employer to ensure, so far as is reasonably practicable, the health, safety and welfare at work of all employees extends to the duty to provide first aid. The duty to provide adequate first aid is specifically dealt with by the Health and Safety (First Aid) Regulations 1981 SI No. 917 supplemented by an Approved Code of Practice revised in 1997.

The aim of the Regulations is to ensure that all people at work are adequately covered, and their flexibility is designed to ensure people in similar work situations are effectively covered to a similar standard. The Regulations lay down three broad duties:

- The duty of the employer to provide first aid.
- The duty of the employer to inform employees of the arrangements made in connection with first aid.
- The duty of the self-employed person to provide first aid equipment.

What provision of first aid will be considered adequate will depend on a number of factors, such as number and distribution of employees/workers, type of work, location of workplace and distance from external medical facilities. The ACOP highlights the duty of the employer to assess the needs appropriate to the workplace, and guidance explains how the provision should be related to the level of risk. Where there is an occupational health service available to the workplace, the risk assessment will often be guided by that specialist team, as will the monitoring of first aiders and first aid points. It is not always the case, however, that occupational health services offer a first aid facility directly, whether or not they are on site. A duty of care is owed by health professionals who provide any form of treatment, including first aid to individuals.

Employers must inform their employees of the arrangements that have been made, including the location of facilities, equipment and personnel. An employer who employs 50 or more people must provide one or more 'suitable persons' to render first aid in the case of injury or illness at work, or at least to take charge of a situation where this becomes necessary. If a first aid room is considered necessary, it should have adequate lighting, heating and ventilation, be clean and large enough to hold a couch and have space for several persons. For more details on the training requirements and occupational health issues of first aid at work, see Chapter 4.

Occupational health perspectives

The Management of Health and Safety at Work Regulations 1999 SI No. 3242 require that employers carry out health surveillance, and specific health surveillance procedures are required under the Control of Substances Hazardous to Health 2002 SI 2677 (COSHH) regulations. These can also include certain screening procedures. These occupational health screenings should not be confused with other general health screening procedures that may be carried out as part of primary health care through the general practitioner, such as cervical smears to help in the detection and prevention of cervical cancer in women, or cholesterol testing for early detection of the risk of heart disease. The focus of this chapter is to consider the employment law implications for the various types of health surveillance required in specific types of workplace hazards in terms of the role of occupational health in undertaking this important aspect of practice.

The first and most significant aspect of health surveillance is the risk assessment of the work processes, as outlined in Chapter 1. Once a risk assessment has been completed, the best methods of control and prevention should be put in place to prevent or reduce the risk – so far as it is reasonably foreseeable and practical – of workers suffering from work-related ill health or injury. It is good practice for management and trade union representatives, with advice from health and safety and occupational health professionals, to be jointly involved in drawing up the necessary policies and procedures and deciding on the best way to reduce the risks. There are employment law obligations to consult staff on health and safety matters. If some form of health surveillance is required – which will depend on the type of hazard and the risk – this will need to determine who and what is meant by the following in any protocols:

- *A responsible person:* such as a suitably trained line manager checking for any reactions, for example by inspecting hands for skin damage when solvents are being used, or using a questionnaire to check for any symptoms or problems.
- *A qualified person:* such as an occupational health practitioner or other health professional undertaking regular tests, for example lung function or hearing tests.

- *Biological monitoring:* such as blood tests to check if there is any take-up of chemicals from exposure, or immunisation results to check, for example, that a hepatitis B vaccine has been effective.
- *Medical surveillance:* a medical examination by a doctor, usually a qualified occupational health physician, which may include a clinical examination for the purposes of assessing exposure to certain chemicals.
- *Keeping health surveillance records:* these records are not about individuals and so should not usually contain confidential clinical information. They should contain general details of past and present history of exposure to the hazard, details of health surveillance procedures regarding fitness to work, restrictions, etc. This may be as simple as keeping a register of who handled a particular chemical, on what date and for how long. The records should be retained for the recommended period (up to 50 years for COSHH records) as they can provide evidence of risk assessment and compliance with safety standards, and also need to be available for inspection by appropriate authorities.

One of the most important aspects of health and safety management is undertaking an adequate risk assessment of working practices to ensure that a safe system of work is in place. This is particularly vital where there is a risk to health as well as safety. Many of the risks to the health of the worker are not seen or felt; in other words, there are no signs or symptoms until the effects have taken hold, perhaps many years later, as for example with exposure to asbestos and the later development of asbestosis or other malignant disease, or hand–arm vibration symptoms including vibration white finger. However, with some jobs the ill effects may be immediate, e.g. working in confined spaces, diving or working in extremes of temperature.

Health screening is only appropriate when certain criteria are met and in valid circumstances, as exampled in the work of Wilson and Jungner. The criteria were developed in 1968 (see Fig. 3.1), and remain as valid today as when first published.

---

(1)   The condition being screened for should be an important health problem.
(2)   The natural history of the condition should be well understood.
(3)   There should be a detectable early stage.
(4)   Treatment should be of more benefit at an early stage than at a later stage.
(5)   A suitable test should be devised for the early stage.
(6)   The test should be acceptable.
(7)   Intervals for repeating the test should be determined.
(8)   Adequate health service provision should be made for the extra clinical workload resulting from screening.
(9)   The risks, both physical and psychological, should be less than the benefits.
(10) The costs should be balanced against the benefits.

Wilson, J.M. & Jungner, G. (1968) *Principles and Practice of Screening for Disease.* World Health Organization, Public Health Paper No. 34, Geneva.

Fig. 3.1   The Wilson and Jungner criteria for appraising the validity of a screening programme.

Some situations make it a requirement under the regulations to carry out health surveillance, but there are other circumstances where health surveillance is necessary as a general health and safety good practice procedure. The HSE suggest the following framework for assessing whether health surveillance is indicated as necessary:[10]

- There is an identifiable disease or adverse health condition related to the work concerned.
- Valid techniques are available to detect indication of the disease or condition.
- There is a reasonable likelihood that the disease or condition may occur under the particular work conditions, and surveillance is likely to further the protection of the health and safety of the employees covered.

It is necessary to consider all these points carefully as some health surveillances, assessments or screenings may be omitted in error, or conducted as a result of custom and practice rather than being based on regulatory requirement, scientific evidence and ethical principles. Any screening procedures that are undertaken as part of health surveillance should be related to the effects of the particular hazard on the health of the employee. It is not an opportunity to undertake procedures that may be invasive, time consuming or costly unless the outcome of any health problems so detected is of direct relevance to the employee's ability and safety in doing the job.

Cooperation and communication

Occupational health should be involved in advising management and health and safety departments on what measures are needed to protect the health of workers, and at times, to advise on safe systems of work. They are often aware of the health and medical history of the individual, which remains confidential information (see Chapter 2) but nonetheless can help to guide safe practices and adjustments. Employers who appoint doctors, nurses or other health professionals to advise them on employee health and health surveillance should ensure that these people are appropriately trained and qualified to provide the necessary expertise in occupational health. Evidence of qualifications and proper registration with a professional body should always be checked.

Occupational health should also be involved, as one of the stakeholders, in the development of relevant and robust policies and procedures for the protection of workers' health in relation to safe systems of working. Of course, the occupational health service will also need to have its own departmental policies and procedures on how health surveillance is to be carried out.

An often overlooked but significant factor that must be detailed in health surveillance protocols is what to do if there is an abnormal health surveillance finding. Some points to consider for inclusion in the policy and procedures are:

- Does the individual require referral?
- Who will pay the cost, and is there a budget?
- Should the individual(s) continue working?

- Who else should be informed?
- Is this a prescribed disease under RIDDOR legislation?
- What confidential issues need to be considered?
- Should the process be stopped?

The next case study in this chapter on page 69 clearly demonstrates how clear policy and procedures can help to deal efficiently and effectively with any problems that arise.

Health surveillance is just one part of the general principles involved in the prevention of work-related ill health, disease and injury. A priority that follows identification of the potential problems through surveillance is for employers to avoid or reduce health risks by combating the problem at source: for example, by providing suitable ventilation for dusts and fumes, or by arranging work so that regular breaks are taken away from the computer workstation or from working in a cold store. Through regular reviews and updates, health surveillance can also identify where there is a breakdown in preventative measures.

The effects of work on health

The effects of work on health can be wide ranging. Advice from an occupational health consultant and treating specialist will be necessary in many situations where there is any significant cause for concern. The Health and Safety Executive uses the expertise of specialists to develop appropriate guidelines. As previously mentioned, the cornerstones of the legislation are duty, practicability and reasonableness. In other words, the employer must act: it is his duty to carry out risk assessments, and to put in place policies, procedures and safe systems of work. The employee then has a duty to follow these policies, procedures and safe systems of work. The procedures must be practical, sensible and reasonable. For example, the wearing of personal protective equipment, such as a respirator or mask when exposed to dust or fumes may not be practical if other measures are available to protect the worker. Respirators and masks are uncomfortable; they require training to wear them, and supervision to ensure they are worn, as well as maintenance and replacement. Wearing them would not necessarily be the most reasonable way to reduce exposure to the hazard when it could be feasible, say, to have local exhaust ventilation instead. Respirators are also a constant financial outlay, while local exhaust ventilation would protect several employees at once and would be a one-off capital outlay (with costs for periodic maintenance). Each worker would also be more comfortable and more able to work efficiently than if he were wearing a respirator.

Once it has been decided, following the risk assessment, that health surveillance is necessary, occupational health services can advise management of the most suitable methods, based on ethical principles. The advice will depend on the type of hazards the workers are exposed to, and these can be categorised under the following broad headings:

- Chemicals and substances including micro-organisms.
- Physical hazards including radiation, manual handling and noise.

- Ergonomics including display screen equipment.
- Mental health.
- Ways of working, including night work, confined spaces; vulnerable adults.

Regulations and health surveillance

Health surveillance for chemicals and substances is governed, as stated, mainly by the Control of Substances Hazardous to Health Regulations 2002 SI No. 2677 (as amended) but some substances have specific legislation or guidance, e.g. lead (Regulation 10 of the Control of Lead at Work Regulations 1998 SI No. 543) and asbestos (Regulation 16 of the Control of Asbestos at Work Regulations 1987 SI No. 2115 as amended by the Control of Asbestos at Work Regulations 2002 SI No. 2675). The HSE guide *Health Surveillance at Work* gives a comprehensive list of other guidance on chemical and biological hazards and health surveillance in the appendices.[11]

The COSHH regulations require employers to prevent or take proper steps, including risk assessments, to control adequately the exposure of their employees, and other persons who may be affected, to hazardous substances. In addition, the regulations require the maintenance, examination and testing of control measures; the provision of information, instruction and training; emergency planning; and, in some cases, exposure monitoring and health surveillance of employees, preparing procedures to deal with accidents, incidents and emergencies involving hazardous substances. In meeting their obligations under COSHH, employers must have regard to the practical advice contained in the COSHH Approved Code of Practice. The Approved Codes of Practice (ACOPs) in relation to health and safety provide guidance on the legal requirements to be met in specific situations, including particular risk assessments to be covered. While guidance has no direct legal enforceability, any failure to comply with guidance in risk assessments and recommended working practice may be evidence of negligence. Although only the courts can give an authoritative interpretation of the law when considering the application of health and safety legislation, the HSE and local authority inspectors expect employers to follow the guidance in the relevant ACOP or be able to demonstrate that any alternative procedures/processes they have used, at variance with the ACOP, can be shown to provide an equivalent level of protection.

Before any decision is made about what form of health surveillance is required, it is necessary to know how the substances enter the body, and how they can affect it. Manufacturers have a duty to provide hazard data sheets giving information, but these may be limited in what they reveal. The Chemicals (Hazard Information and Packaging for Supply) Regulations 2002 SI No. 1689, also known as CHIP3, is the law that applies to suppliers of dangerous chemicals. Its purpose is to protect people and the environment from the effects of those chemicals by requiring suppliers to provide information about the dangers, and to package them safely. It applies to most chemicals, but not all.

CHIP requires the supplier of a dangerous chemical to:

- Identify the hazards (dangers) of the chemical. This is known as 'classification'.
- Give information about the hazards to their customers. Suppliers usually provide this information on the package itself (e.g. on a label) and, if supplied for use at work, in a safety data sheet (SDS).
- Package the chemical safely.

Health surveillance for physical hazards

Specific legislation exists giving guidance on health surveillance for several physical hazards.

Ionising Radiations Regulations 1999 SI No. 3232 (IRR99)

These require that anyone working with ionising radiation has regular, periodic health surveillance by an appointed doctor. This will commence at pre-employment to assess fitness to undertake the work. Periodic review may then be by questionnaire completed by the employee. The appointed doctor will then review the questionnaire together with:

- The employee's medical file
- Dosimeter records over the last 12 months
- Details of any sickness absence

The doctor or an occupational health nurse may then see the employee to discuss any health issues and the employee will have his health record signed to continue working.

The Control of Noise at Work Regulations 2005 SI No. 1643

These came into force from April 2006, with a two-year transitional period for the music and entertainment industry until 6 April 2008. Noise Induced Hearing Loss or NIHL is one of the most prevalent, irreversible industrial diseases. Health surveillance alone will not prevent it from occurring. It is necessary to follow a complete hearing protection programme, using risk assessment, noise reduction and control of exposure measures such as changing work patterns, restricting access to noisy areas, etc.

Where control measures reduce exposure to below the action levels, no extensive health surveillance might be necessary. However, if control measures cannot eliminate the health risk then hearing tests should be undertaken at the start of employment to give a base line audiogram with subsequent regular hearing checks, generally annually for the first two years of employment and subsequently three-yearly unless any abnormality is noted or exposure to noise is extremely high. The audiograms can be carried out by someone who understands the audiometric data, such as a trained audiometrician, or a doctor or nurse with the appropriate training and experience. Further details and comprehensive guidance on health surveillance for noise will be found in HSE booklet *Controlling Noise at Work L108*.

A comprehensive hearing conservation programme should also ensure that the employee understands:

- The results of any hearing tests or health checks.
- The significance of any hearing damage.
- The assessment in writing of his hearing.
- What happens if any abnormality is detected.
- Where to seek further medical advice and referral to his GP.
- That proper records will be kept (see Chapter 2).
- That his hearing protection must fit correctly, and how to maintain it.
- The importance of following the company hearing conservation programme.

Control of Vibration at Work Regulations 2005 SI No. 1093

Exposure to vibrations which may cause hand–arm vibration syndrome (HAVS) is now governed by the above regulations and there are interim guidelines for health surveillance in line with the European Directives. This HSE guidance indicates that health surveillance should be offered to employees who are regularly exposed above the 'action values' of 2.5 m/s^2 A(8), to those who are occasionally exposed, and to those who already are suffering from 'hand–arm vibration syndrome'. Training to undertake HAVS health surveillance is formulated by the Faculty of Occupational Medicine. Currently the HSE are recommending a tiered approach to health surveillance so that:

- A qualified person, such as an occupational health nurse, can make enquiries about symptoms and carry out clinical assessment of HAVS; whilst
- An occupational health physician will carry out clinical examination and formal diagnosis as well as advise on fitness to work.

It must be remembered that any screening or physical examination undertaken should only be related to the condition that may result from exposure to vibration, such as HAVS or Raynaud's phenomena, and this can include:

- Relevant work history and related medical history.
- Physical examination of relevant affected parts, or potentially affected parts.
- Investigations, such as MRI.

Health surveillance for whole body vibration is provided in the HSE booklet *Control of Back Pain Risks from Whole Body Vibration: Advice for Employers on the Control of Vibration at Work Regulations, 2005*. The advice suggests that employers:

- Carry out a risk assessment.
- Know how and to whom back symptoms should be reported.
- Have an annual questionnaire check list.
- Have access or referral to an occupational health service.

Manual Handling Operations Regulations 1992 SI No. 2793 (as amended)

These Regulations require that an employee is physically suitable to carry out manual handling operations. This is also dealt with in Chapter 1, covering the recruitment and pre-employment considerations. No specific continuing health surveillance is required beyond management properly training staff and being aware of the capabilities required of their employees to continue to undertake manual handling tasks, as provided in MHSWR. Proper and timely reviews after any sickness absence episodes that may be linked to manual handling related injury should be followed up as a matter of good practice.

Divers

Health surveillance for diving at work must be carried out by a medical examiner approved by the Health and Safety Executive. The standards required are based on both physical and psychological fitness to dive, as prescribed by the Diving at Work Regulations 1997 SI No. 2776 as there are certain medical conditions that would normally be a contraindication for diving. Medical requirements for fitness to dive will differ according to the reason for diving. It is advisable that people first seek general health advice from their GP before embarking on a diving career and before proceeding to the full preliminary medical examination by the authorised initial medical examiner. After the preliminary medical examination, annual medical assessment is required by an approved doctor.

The Work at Heights Regulations 2005 SI No. 735

The Regulations cover all the safety aspects of working in these specific areas as there is a higher risk of accidents, with preventative steps to avoid them in place. Workers who work at heights should be assessed for their fitness to undertake this work following a risk assessment. Again, the main aspect of working at heights is safety and following a safe system of work. However, workers should be agile and mobile enough to deal with situations at a height and this will require an assessment of their neurological and musculoskeletal systems. The Health and Safety Executive say that studies showing common situations where falls from height occur demonstrate that these events are usually due to poor management control rather than equipment failure.

The Confined Spaces Regulations 1997 SI No. 1713

These cover working in confined spaces such as storage tanks, silos, sewers where there is danger from a lack of oxygen or from toxic fumes, gases or vapours. In terms of health surveillance, workers should be assessed for any tendency towards claustrophobia and for their general fitness to wear breathing apparatus and respirators.

Vulnerable persons

There are some persons who are or may be more vulnerable to health and safety risks at work, and these include:

- young persons
- new and expectant mothers
- some disabled persons
- older workers

Night workers

Under the Working Time Regulations 1998 SI No. 1833, employers must offer night workers a free health assessment before they start working nights and on a regular basis while they are working nights. In many cases it will be appropriate to do this once a year, though employers can offer a health assessment more than once a year if they feel it is necessary, depending on the work and the risk assessment for the work. Workers do not have to take up the opportunity to have a health assessment, but it must be offered by the employer. The health assessment can be made up of two parts:

- a questionnaire
- an examination by an appropriately qualified doctor or nurse

The latter is only necessary if the employer has doubts about the worker's fitness for night work.

The health assessment should take into account the type of work and the risk assessment. If a worker suffers from problems that are caused or made worse by night work, the employer should transfer him to day work if possible. A record of the name of the night worker, when an assessment was offered (and when he had the assessment, if there was one) and the result of any assessment must be kept for at least two years.

Where the type of work may be hazardous to other people

Generally, where the work is hazardous to other people it is also hazardous to the worker. However, there are situations where the safety of the public must be paramount, and driving and flying are two examples. Both are covered by legislation other than general health and safety and employment law.

- The UK's Civil Aviation Authority (CAA) follows guidelines for statutory medical assessments from the European Union's Joint Aviation Authority for aircrew and air traffic controllers. The CAA website provides full details of the medical checks and certification requirements: www.caa.co.uk.

There are several different types of vehicles that are driven in a working situation including:

- cars or vans
- minibus carrying 9–16 people
- passenger-carrying vehicles, such as a buses or coaches
- LGV and HGV – long or heavy goods vehicles
- cranes
- forklift trucks
- tractors and farm implements

The health surveillance required will depend on the type of vehicle. Both the DVLA and the HSE give guidance on the different areas requiring health surveillance and the general statutory obligations relating to driving regulations. In the HSE guidance *Driving at Work* (2003), it is recommended that employers satisfy themselves that their drivers are fit and healthy to drive safely, so as not to put themselves or others at risk. They should ask the following questions:

- Do drivers of heavy lorries, for whom there are statutory requirements for medical examination, have the appropriate medical certification?
- When are health checks appropriate for drivers?
- Should staff who drive at work be reminded that they must satisfy the eyesight requirements set out in the Highway Code?
- Are drivers aware that they should not drive while taking a course of medication that might impair their judgement?

Where required, regular health checks or medical examinations should include:

- Relevant work history and related medical history. There are certain conditions that exclude people from holding a driving licence, and the medical examiner will be aware of the DVLA requirements for different categories of driver/licence.
- Physical examination will include:
  - ○ eyesight test, including visual fields and vestibular function
  - ○ ears, including hearing and vestibular function
  - ○ blood pressure
  - ○ neurological and musculoskeletal system checks

Occupational health action

The Management of Health and Safety at Work Regulations 1999 SI No. 3242 require that suitable health surveillance is undertaken for young persons and new and expectant mothers, and again this will also depend on the risk assessment covering the work they do: Regulations 16–19 deal specifically with these groups.

Health surveillance can also apply to disabled persons, and here the Disability Discrimination Act 1995 should also be considered because fitness to work must be based on the criteria for the particular job. Health and safety at work applies to everyone and is the overriding issue in all cases. Consideration must be given as to whether working practices or equipment can be modified for workers – in other words, can the work be made to fit the workers, rather than the worker to fit the work.

Recent research[12] indicates that there are some myths and misconceptions regarding age and health status, and so care should be taken in requiring additional health surveillance of one group of people as against another for age-related reasons. Any such selective surveillance or screening programmes could be discriminatory unless they can be proven to be objectively indicated, for example by the risk assessment or statutory requirement. This research found that older workers are a valuable resource for organisations and that their general health, cognitive capacity, sensory ability, strength and endurance were not necessarily impaired because of age. The simple measures that can be used to improve functioning and productivity of workers are right for any age group, not just the older worker.

Working with chemicals and hazardous substances

Where chemicals and other potentially hazardous substances are used in the workplace, health surveillance is vital. It is known that chemicals and substances enter the body in four ways:

- inhalation
- ingestion
- injection
- in through the skin (absorption)

Inhalation

Chemicals and substances including micro-organisms can affect the body by being inhaled into the respiratory system, and in the lungs they may cross into the bloodstream. They come in numerous forms including dust, fumes, gases, vapours and particles. Some, such as hydrogen cyanide gas, can have an immediate lethal effect, while others, such as asbestos, take many years to develop health effects. Health effects may occur with longer-term exposure to respiratory sensitisers, which can cause (occupational) asthma, a debilitating disease that can sometimes end a person's career. In such cases employees are likely to be covered by disability legislation.

The BOHR[13] list of most frequently reported agents for causing allergy is given in Fig. 3.2 and a list of occupations in Fig. 3.3.

Isocyanates in paints and foams
Flour and grain dust
Colophony and fluxes
Latex
Animals
Aldehydes
Work dusts

Fig. 3.2   Most frequently reported agents causing asthma (BOHRF, 2004)[13].

Bakers	Storage workers
Food processors	Farm workers
Forestry workers	Waiters
Chemical workers	Cleaners
Plastics and rubber workers	Painters
Metal workers	Plastics workers
Welders	Dental workers
Textile workers	Laboratory technicians
Electrical & electronic production workers	

Fig. 3.3   Who is most at risk from developing asthma? (BOHRF, 2004)[13].

Health surveillance will depend on the scientific evidence of the effect of the particular substance, and then the priority for the employer must be taking steps, based on the evidence and health surveillance, to control exposure in the working environment by methods such as local exhaust ventilation and safe handling procedures. Once suitable ventilation and safe systems of work are in place, further health surveillance will be necessary.

The surveillance of people handling inhaled substances likely to cause occupational asthma will start on their appointment to the job that carries the risk and continue throughout their exposure/employment. Depending on the type of substance and length of exposure, and the control measures in place, this may be by:

(1) *Questionnaire:* this could be all that is necessary periodically, usually annually, depending on exposure. A sample questionnaire is given at Appendix 3.
(2) *Lung function testing (LFT):* a base-line LFT is undertaken and the frequency of further tests will depend on exposure and comments made on the periodic questionnaire. This is usually carried out more frequently in the first two years of employment.
(3) *Review by an occupational health nurse or doctor:* all periodic questionnaires and LFTs will be reviewed by the nurse or doctor, who will decide if and when further action is needed.

Anyone developing symptoms of asthma, or rhinitis, should be seen more frequently and, to assist the diagnosis, peak flow meter reading should be taken four times a day for three weeks. Then they should be referred to a consultant occupational health or respiratory physician.

Case study

A 25-year-old female researcher was working towards a PhD in an area of research related to cardiac tissue. The cardiac tissue was obtained from rats, and the researcher was required to work in an animal facility, which contained predominately mice and rats, for 25–30 hours a week in order to harvest the tissue. She had been suffering from rhinitis and conjunctivitis for two months, but she had attributed these symptoms to a succession of colds and occasional bouts of hay fever. The symptoms came to the attention of the university's occupational health service when she completed her annual surveillance questionnaire with them.

Her lung function tests of FEV1 and FVC were showing some reduction on previous readings, and she revealed on enquiry that she occasionally felt a little breathless when she had been working in the animal facility for extended periods. Blood was taken for testing for IgE serology specific to rat urine and dander and mouse urine and dander. Attendance in the animal house was then restricted to ten hours a week and advice was given on the use of respiratory protective equipment (RPE), and a positive pressure air-fed hood was provided for this purpose.

The results received three weeks later showed that the researcher in question had become highly sensitive to rat urine and dander, and moderately sensitive to mouse

Cont.

urine. The sensitivity to rat was so high that a decision was made by the occupational physician that any further exposure had the potential to be life threatening.

After making the researcher aware of the results and the potential risk, it was mutually agreed that under no circumstances could she continue with the research project. After discussion she changed direction for her PhD and joined another project group not working with animals.

Within the university in question, all true cases of occupational asthma in the previous 24 months (four in total) had been initially identified by questionnaire. Spirometry is not performed in isolation because of the possibility of frequent false positives as a result of poor respiratory technique.

Ingestion

It is often felt that the majority of substances which enter the body via ingestion do so because of such factors as unsafe systems of work, poor personal hygiene and habits, incorrect labelling of containers, and people not washing their hands after visiting the lavatory or before eating meals. COSHH regulations require that where substances hazardous to health are handled no eating, drinking, smoking or applying of cosmetics should take place. Occupational health can help by reinforcing knowledge and good practice relating to these factors with both management and workers. This is of particular importance for employees in areas where micro-organisms are a hazard, such as health care workers, water industry workers, farmers and animal handlers. Immunisations may be required as part of health surveillance for some of these workers.

Travel broadens the mind but it can also lead to broadened problems relating to health. Employees who have to travel abroad as part of their job may be exposed to biological hazards that can be ingested, especially if, for example, their work takes them to rural areas in developing countries. Therefore advice should be sought from bodies such as the National Travel Health Network and Centre (NaTHNaC). For information on which immunisations may be needed and what extra advice is required to be given, see www.nathnac.org or phone the advice line for health professionals on 0845 602 6712. Some companies with frequent travellers either have their own specialist occupational health teams who are appropriately trained and qualified to advise, or buy in to one of the private organisations offering specific advice for travellers.

Injection

The commonest example of injection of a hazardous substance occurs with health care workers and accidental inoculation by 'needle stick injury', where there is a risk of their acquiring a blood-borne virus infection. Over the years, moves have been made to introduce safer systems of handling sharps in health care. Health surveillance of health care workers includes ensuring that they have had suitable immunisations, such as hepatitis B, when these are available. The blood-borne viruses of hepatitis B and C have both short- and long-term effects. At present there is no immunisation for hepatitis C. The occupational health surveillance of those involved with exposure-prone procedures will need to follow the latest guidelines issued by the Department of Health and the Health and Safety Executive.

There is also a risk of accidental injection for certain other occupations, such as prison officers, customs officers, and emergency services. A safe system of work is essential, but the risk remains and should be mitigated to its lowest level.

For people who work overseas in rural areas or developing countries, or those who work with exotic animals, there is always a risk of disease, bites and stings. Specific health surveillance of overseas workers can involve the unusual and unexpected in order to prevent injected toxins and micro-organisms. Malaria is singularly the most important hazard to the tropical traveller with up to 30,000 North American and European travellers contracting malaria annually.[14] Therefore health surveillance may be required from occupational health both before and after travel. The National Travel Health Network and Centre provides an advice line for health professionals who have queries about travel scenarios that involve either complex itineraries or travellers with special health needs: see www.nathnac.org or phone the advice line for health professionals on 0845 602 6712.

Absorption or in through the skin

Dermatitis is one of the most common work-related health problems. It is the reaction of the skin to penetration through the barrier layer by a substance that causes inflammation. It may be caused by contact with any substance, even water, depending on what systems of work are in place: for example, frequent hand-washing without adequate drying facilities and suitable skin moisturisers can cause dermatitis in susceptible individuals. There are many substances that are known to cause a reaction, and some substances that are known irritants or sensitisers; these are listed in HSE Guidance note MS 24, though it should be noted that the HSE make it clear that even their list is not exhaustive.

Where the risk assessment has identified that the worker(s) are exposed to substances likely to cause skin problems, health surveillance is necessary. This may be by the provision of information and training to enable employees to undertake their own skin inspection and report any abnormalities to the responsible person, who may be an experienced manager, trained by occupational health; alternatively, they may be reported directly to occupational health. Records of this health surveillance must be kept in accordance with other COSHH related records – see also Chapter 2.

There are other health problems caused by absorption of substances, such as cutting oils that can cause acne, and organophosphates (OPs), which are the most toxic of pesticides. The latter are used as insecticides in agriculture and horticulture, and are the basis for poisonous substances such as sarin.

OPs are a good example of how a chemical can be absorbed through the skin and cause severe health problems, both acute and chronic. They act by inhibiting the enzymes that break down the neurotransmitter acetylcholine so that its level rises at nerve synapses and neuromuscular junctions. Farmers or workers using OP dips regularly should seek advice on health surveillance from a medical

Case study: food processing

Company A had employees experiencing irritant contact dermatitis. The company handled cooked meat joints. These were sliced, and then packed into small plastic packs, which were heat sealed and packed into cartons for supply to a supermarket chain. Initial investigation by the health and safety officer revealed that no hazardous substances were in use. However, the working environment was very cold (3–5 °C), with low relative humidity, around 20%. The workers wore single-use vinyl gloves for most of the day and were required to wash their hands frequently (typically between 15 and 20 times each day) using a skin cleanser containing a high level of active anti-microbial. Water temperature for hand-washing was around 45 °C. No aftercare hand cream was available.

An assessment of the situation by a dermatological expert suggested that it was this combination that was responsible for the dermatitis. Low temperature and low relative humidity are well known to cause damage to the skin as a barrier. The hyperhydration occurring underneath the occlusive gloves was equivalent to wet work. The skin cleanser was unnecessarily aggressive and the water temperature too high.

Action

(1)　It was felt that the use of occlusive gloves was excessive. Their use was limited to those – relatively brief – occasions when the meat was actually handled while being placed into the slicing machine. Once in the machine, there was no hand contact. This significantly reduced the hyperhydration that had been occurring.

(2)　The use of an anti-microbial cleanser was limited to use when entering the workplace and when the hands were heavily soiled with organic matter. A suitably buffered alcohol sanitising rub was recommended for more general use. The buffering effect actually resulted in a build-up of moisturiser in the skin, such that the workforce had to wash their hands occasionally so as to avoid a 'sticky' feeling.

(3)　Water temperature was reduced to lukewarm to avoid damage to skin, thus helping to maintain the skin's natural barrier.

(4)　An emollient (moisturising) lotion was provided for use when leaving the work area so as to replace the natural oils in the skin lost during the working period.

(5)　A programme of skin health surveillance was introduced to detect damaged skin before this could develop into full-scale irritant contact dermatitis.

These actions were sufficient to eliminate any further outbreaks and to allow those whose skin had been damaged to return to work once their skin had healed.

practitioner who is familiar with the risks of the process and understands the principles of health surveillance. This might include sampling for cholinesterase measurement before the dipping season, and repeat sampling if adverse effects or significant accidental exposures occur. Urine sampling for OP metabolites, as a measure of exposure, may be a useful additional way of monitoring the effectiveness of control measures. More details will be found in the HSE guidance *Biological monitoring of workers exposed to organophosphates* MS 17 1987 and on the website of the Health Protection Agency: www.hpa.org.uk.

Business travel and health surveillance

Business travel today covers a wide range of circumstances and there are many reasons for travelling abroad, such as to attend meetings and conferences, or to undertake research. Travel may often be on a regular basis for journalists, relief NGO (non-governmental organisation, e.g. Red Cross or Red Crescent) workers, the diplomatic services and those who work in the travel industry itself. Employers have a duty of care to their employees while they are travelling or working abroad, which is covered in the employment law sections in Chapter 4.

The hazards travellers may be exposed to are wide and varied. The importance of risk assessment cannot be stressed enough here.

- Where will they be travelling to?
- How will they be travelling?
- Where will they be staying?
- What will they be doing?
- How long will they be doing it for?
- What health facilities are available in the area?

Therefore in order to comply with the duty of care the employers should ensure that their employee health surveillance includes:

- Ensuring that they are fit to travel: medical and dental care issues are both vital.
- Ensuring that overseas work will suit an individual's health needs, i.e. that they have the physical and psychological ability to cope, and that any existing medical condition will not be made worse by the work.
- Offering immunisations, malarial prophylaxis and general advice on preventative measures against illness and injury.
- Providing suitable medical kits/equipment, e.g. sharps, needles and syringes for travel to certain areas.
- Ensuring access to medical care for employees working overseas.
- Offering appropriate follow-up health review upon return.

Where postings abroad are a known factor of the job, the employment contract should reflect the terms applicable. This might include the expectation for the employee to have required vaccinations as necessary for travel to particular countries. Employers must, however, bear in mind that circumstances and people's health change over time. Any objections an employee has to vaccinations or other medications should be considered on an individual basis. If there is any conflict or risk, expert advice should be sought and reasonable adjustments made where appropriate.

There is the concept of informed choice, which is also to be considered. Certain jobs in certain locations are inherently dangerous. A classic example would be that of the war correspondent reporting news from inside a dangerous country. A risk assessment is essential to the informed choice process. It would not be good practice for an employer to force a posting upon someone who chose not to take a posting into a country known to be high risk and dangerous. The risk assessment factors will highlight training and information needs, such as the starting point, as standard, of the Foreign Office web site (www.fco.gov.uk), or the National Travel Health and Network and Centre (www.nathnac.org, or phone their advice line 0845 602 6712), or one of the commercial organisations that offer these services. Personal security, cultural and gender advice with regard to country-specific training can also be provided from both in-house resources and external specialist organisations.

Working abroad takes people away from accustomed services and recognised personal and social security systems. Employees should be advised to be wise as to health risks and considerations when travelling, working or posted abroad. Employers should:

- Take Foreign and Commonwealth Office advice about the country to which employees are travelling.
- Carry out a risk assessment, inform employees of any known risks and give advice to reduce exposure to them.
- Obtain informed consent to travel or be posted to dangerous locations.
- Check on necessary vaccinations or other precautions for safeguarding health, including taking a medical kit if sterilisation or cross-infection are potential risks.
- Maintain personal safety as a top priority.
- Make sure people know where colleagues are at all times.
- Advise staff to have transport back-up and a contact telephone number for a recognised taxi service.
- Be aware of local customs and laws concerning alcohol, clothing, behaviour, etc.: some countries have zero tolerance for alcohol and driving.
- If a situation is dangerous, give advice as to planning what to do when faced with danger: e.g. shout, make a fuss and make people aware that someone feels threatened.
- Try to ensure that staff are aware of mobile phone network for emergency use.
- Advise of the contact details of the British Consulate.
- Be clear about insurance cover: tell employees what the company is covering – for example, health insurance, life insurance – and advise them of what the employer is not covering – family insurance, off-duty and other exclusions, for example.

Summary

The examples of health surveillance given in this chapter are not exhaustive; they serve as an example of good practice guidelines. Employers and occupational health professionals can seek further advice and help on specific hazards from the Health and Safety Executive guidance and codes of practice, many of which can be downloaded free of charge from the internet.

In summary, then:

- Health surveillance depends on the risk assessment for the job.
- Health surveillance is the last-stop check that can show up when other control measures are not adequate or where failures and problems are not otherwise revealed.

- Health surveillance should be relevant to the work undertaken.
- It is not ethical to use health surveillance as a means of diagnosing other, unrelated, health problems.

References

1. Department for Work and Pensions (2004) *Building Capacity for work: A UK Framework for Vocational Rehabilitation*. DWP.
2. Health and Safety Executive (1999) *Health Surveillance at Work*. HSE, London.
3. Civil Aviation Authority. The CAA also authorises medical examiners.
4. Docks Regulations 1988 SI No. 1655.
5. Section 5, Health and Safety at Work etc. Act 1974.
6. Corporate Manslaughter Bill 2005.
7. As reported by the Health and Safety Executive, 11 October 2005, www.hse.gov.uk.
8. Example provided by Linda Goldman, BDS, LL.B, Barrister. Chambers of Bernard Pearl, 7 New Square, Lincoln's Inn, London.
9. HSE Books, Form B1510.
10. Health and Safety Executive (1999) *Management of Health and Safety at Work: Approved Code of Practice and Guidance*. HSE, London.
11. Health and Safety Executive (1999) *Health Surveillance at Work* HSG61. HSE, London.
12. Health and Safety Executive (2005) *Facts and Misconceptions about Age, Health Status and Employability*. HSE Report: HSL/2005/20.
13. British Occupational Health Research Foundation (2004) *Occupational Asthma: A Guide For Employers, Workers and Their Representatives*. BOHRF, London.
14. Lobel, H. O. & Kozarsk, P. E. (1997) Update on prevention of malaria in travellers. *Journal of the American Medical Association* (Dec) **278**: 1767–71.

Chapter 4
Occupational Health Services

Introduction of occupational health

People's health has been affected by their work for hundreds of years. There is evidence that slaves in Egyptian times covered their mouths with material to prevent themselves from inhaling the dust from mining the stones used to build the pyramids. Over the centuries it has been accepted that some occupations are responsible for the morbidity and mortality of the workers. Ramazzini (see Chapter 1) first described a range of occupational diseases, including the writer's cramp suffered by scribes and clerks working long hours in offices. This is now referred to as a work-related upper limb disorder, and is still prevalent today with the introduction of computer terminals into offices and on to desk tops and tables not designed for the purpose.

One has only to read the novels of Dickens, such as *Hard Times*, and picture the conditions people were working and living under in the nineteenth century to appreciate that these may well have contributed to poor health and accidents. At that time children were employed from a young age, when not yet fully grown, so that not only communicable diseases but deformity and early death were rife. The industrial revolution in Great Britain in the eighteenth and nineteenth centuries led to some wealthy and benevolent factory owners – often Quaker families –, employing factory doctors. In the latter part of the nineteenth century Colman's Mustard employed what has been now been recognised as the first occupational health nurse, Phillipa Flowerday. Although in those days there was no registration for nurses and certainly no specialist fields of nursing practice, Miss Flowerday was a trained nurse who worked in the surgery in the morning and then visited the sick workers and their families in their homes in the afternoon. The specialist fields of industrial medicine and nursing, later called occupational health, were to follow in the twentieth century. Certainly from the nursing perspective, this happened following a meeting of the International Congress of Nurses in 1937.[1]

So from the industrial revolution and the advent of factories, and the mechanisation of what were previously manual tasks, came a whole raft of new industrial diseases, many described by Dr Charles Thackrah in 1831 in his book *The Effects of the Principal Arts, Trades and Professions on Health*. He stated that a 'study of medicine which disregards the prevention of disease, limits its ability and honours'.

From those days of the industrial revolution eventually grew the branch of health care and public health known as occupational health. However, it has remained in private hands and was not included as part of the provision of the National Health Service (NHS) from its inception on 5 July 1948. Consequently, to this day the provision of occupational health services remains ad hoc, with a diverse provision to the workers of the United Kingdom and, more recently, the European Union. The UK government announced in October 2005 that it was to appoint a Director of Occupational Health whose role would be to lead the strategy for health and well-being of working age people.[2]

This chapter aims to explore the different types of occupational health provision in the UK today, the role and functions of an occupational health service, and the relevant legal and employment law issues.

Role and function of occupational health

Companies that manufacture products or offer services are clear that these functions are its main business, and therefore its business management priority. For example, if a company makes cars, then producing and selling good quality cars is its prime function. It is not unreasonable to suggest that the health and welfare of its employees is perhaps of secondary concern. The company may not make the connection that a healthy, happy workforce works more effectively and efficiently than an unhealthy, unhappy workforce, but this will need to be made evident through a sound business case analysis to justify the concept and the cost of action. The main aim of the business is more often than not 'maximum output for minimum outlay', in order to prosper and survive. The function of an occupational health service today is to help and support management in achieving that aim. In fulfilling its role, occupational health must consider moral and ethical issues, and at the same time give due consideration to financial and legal matters: a three-stranded approach.

Moral and ethical aspects of occupational health

The work should do the worker no harm: the ethic of 'do unto others as you would have them do unto you'. This ethic has been more recently enshrined in the Declaration of Human Rights,[3] which uses the term 'favourable conditions at work', and in the UK's Human Rights Act 1998. Whether the declarations and legislation are effective is an issue for debate, but certainly a moral responsibility rests upon employers and managers, and for occupational health professionals there is also an ethical responsibility. The employer who does not take care of the health and safety of his workforce could cut corners, put people at risk, sell his product or services at a cheaper rate and, therefore, make more money for himself or for the shareholders – so much so that legislation is in place in the UK to force employers to adhere to health and safety standards.

Some years ago, at a business conference, a group of employers stated that they could not afford to put in place noise controls until there was legislation forcing them to do so because other companies that did not do so would be able to sell their products more cheaply. Noise legislation was passed a few years later. That said, the global labour market now has work done in manufacturing premises and call centres in countries where there is little or no health and safety protection.

The moral and ethical dilemmas continue to present challenges to employers, workers and consumers.

Development of occupational health related law

The first piece of industrial legislation in this country was The Health and Morals of Apprentices Act of 1802, which introduced restrictions on employers sending small boys up chimneys to clean them. Over the next 150 years a variety of Acts were passed on different occupations and premises, covering work in shops, offices, factories, railways and various sectors of work. In the late 1960s the government of the day asked Lord Robens to review the provisions for the health and safety of people at work and other members of the public who could be affected by the work. It is from the report of this review that the overarching Health and Safety at Work etc. Act 1974 (HASWA) was passed. It was and remains a significant piece of legislation as it places responsibility firmly on the employer to 'ensure, as far as is reasonably practicable, the health, safety and welfare at work of his employees'. With this and the current Factories Act, there was considered to be a new era in the management of health and safety at work.

The HASWA also has provision for subordinate legislation, through statutory instruments to be made for specific reasons that have now subsumed and enlarged the functions of the old Factories Acts. These currently include the Management of Health and Safety at Work Regulations 1999 (MHSWR), with their overarching emphasis on prevention through risk assessments. Since the UK joined the European Union (EU), further health and safety regulations have been put in place in order to comply with EU directives.

Many of the HSE guidance notes or ACOPs refer to occupational health services but to date there is no UK legislation that requires an employer to provide any occupational health service. Instead, there are recommendations from various government departments that all employees should have access to occupational health services. Leading companies recognise the value of the occupational health service provision and provide access to the services for their workers.

Combined with health and safety legislation is the growth in employment legislation. These two together mean that to keep a healthy, contented workforce and to comply with legal obligations requires health advice and support from appropriately trained professionals. This can be found through a professional occupational health service.

Financial issues

If the moral reasons for providing occupational health services are not regarded as cost effective, there is the risk of litigation and the costs associated with breaching the law to consider. Sometimes health and safety services are seen as the key to keeping the HSE and other enforcement agencies from prosecuting employers who have failed to make adequate health and safety provisions. Legislation for specific hazards, such as chemical and biological substances, ionising radiation, asbestos and lead, require health surveillance (see Chapter 3), and this involves the work of occupational health specialists. We will discuss the place of the different roles and professions later in this chapter.

With the advent of work systems that are less (physically) hazardous than historical manual work, we see today the rise in stress-related ill health replacing some of the more prevalent and traditional physical health problems of manual workers. There are a wide range of workplace conditions in which there is a need for a whole range of occupational health professionals to advise and support employers and managers on complying with health and safety legislation and other aspects of employment law.

The Chartered Institute of Personnel and Development recently stated that forward-thinking organisations through 'investment in people can achieve excellence and maintain a leading edge', and they recommended promoting a concept of wellness in the workplace.[4] The government's 'Better Routes Task Force' report[5] recommends promoting better management of occupational health and asks that the HSE do more about informing employers of the tax provisions that are available for such things as health screening, counselling, and dealing with work-related conditions and accidents: www.hse.gov.uk/pubns/taxrules.pdf. The same document goes on to suggest that companies that manage their risks to health should be charged lower insurance premiums, and this does occur already in some instances. Case studies on reducing sickness absence, and thereby sickness absence costs, published by the Chartered Institute of Personnel and Development and the Confederation of British Industry[6] serve to illustrate that substantial cost savings can be made and positively recommend the involvement of occupational health in reducing sickness absence (see Chapter 5).

Employers often say that they are covered by insurance so there is no need for them to invest more money in managing health and safety and occupational health. However, the Health and Safety Executive say that for every £1 covered by insurance a further £10 is not covered. Costs not covered by insurance include:

- sick pay
- damage or loss of product or materials
- repairs to plant and equipment
- overtime and temporary labour costs
- production delays
- investigation time
- fines

Functions of an occupational health service

If the moral, legal and financial elements demonstrate that an organisation should have access to an occupational health service, then that organisation will need to be clear what it expects from the service. The World Health Organization (WHO) has stated that although the responsibility for workers' health remains with the employer, the occupational health services will give expert advice to the employer, workers and their representatives. [7] The functions of the service provision should, according to WHO, aim towards:

- Establishing and maintaining a healthy and safe work environment.
- Maintaining a well performing and motivated workforce.
- Preventing of work-related disease and accidents.
- Maintaining and promoting the work ability of workers.

In order to achieve this, occupational health services should offer organisations a range of activities to help, support and advise management. Functions of occupational health services include:[8]

(1) Identification and assessment of the health risk in the workplace.
(2) Surveillance of work environment factors and work practices that affect workers' health.
(3) Participation in the development of programmes for the improvement of working practices, as well as testing and evaluating health aspects of new equipment.
(4) Advice on planning and organisation of work, and design of workplaces.
(5) Advice on occupational health, safety and hygiene, ergonomics and individual and collective protective equipment.
(6) Surveillance of workers' health in relation to work.
(7) Promotion of the adaptation of work to the worker.
(8) Collaboration in providing information, training and education in the fields of occupational health, hygiene and ergonomics.
(9) Contribution to the measures of vocational rehabilitation.
(10) Organisation of first aid and emergency treatment.
(11) Participation in the analysis of occupational accidents and occupational diseases.

All this can only be achieved by suitably trained occupational health specialists working together as part of a team, in cooperation with other management services and using appropriate communications. This book aims to help with the communication processes by giving relevant advice and offering some practical and user-friendly templates for letters, forms, etc., but nothing replaces the occupational health personnel visiting the workplace and working environment, and knowing the premises, equipment and processes the employees are dealing with. Some work is not best conducted from a remote location, such as an office or surgery or computer email system.

Employers and occupational health services should regard the working environment as based on the following four key areas:

- *Premises:* the building or area in which the work is carried out.
- *Plant:* the equipment or machinery used in undertaking the task.
- *Process:* what the worker actually does with, on or to the equipment.
- *People:* the workers or other people who may be involved or affected by the process.

Occupational health professionals

A list of the specialised occupational health professionals who undertake occupational health services was given in Chapter 1, and each of these will now be discussed in more detail. Each discipline plays a different role: many overlap, and all need to work together as part of the occupational health team. All of the health professions in the NHS are regulated by the Council for the Regulation of Health Care Professions, set up under the NHS Reform and Health Care Professions Act 2002.

Occupational health physicians

Occupational medicine is the branch of clinical medicine most active in the field of occupational health. Its principal role is the provision of health advice to organisations and individuals. Occupational physicians must have a wide knowledge of clinical medicine and be competent in a number of important areas. To this end, there are several levels of specialist training that a qualified doctor can undertake, depending on which aspect of occupational health he wishes to be involved in.

For example, a general practitioner may wish to offer specialist services to local companies as part of his GP work, in which case the basic level of qualification might be the Diploma in Occupational Medicine. This will enable him to understand the main issues affecting health and work. Further advancement to become an associate member of the Faculty of Occupational Medicine will be made by studying an agreed training programme to receive a mid training qualification. This is aimed at doctors interested in pursuing a full-time career in occupational medicine and demonstrates their core knowledge in occupational medicine theory and practice. To obtain consultant status in occupational medicine or Membership of the Faculty of Occupational Medicine requires that doctors achieve the Higher Specialist Training by undertaking accredited courses, and that their completed dissertation has been accepted.[9] Full details of the training and experience requirements for the specialty of occupational medicine are available from the Faculty of Occupational Medicine of the Royal College of Physicians.

Occupational health nurses

Occupational health nurses are probably the biggest group of occupational health professionals in the UK. Occupational health has been a specialist branch of nursing for over 70 years and the specialist training today is at first degree level, with many practitioners moving to higher degrees and even doctorates. Fifteen universities in the UK offer courses for occupational health nursing to registered nurses, usually with a minimum of one year's post registration experience. The Nursing and Midwifery Council (NMC) has recently revised the registration of occupational health nurses on to what is now known as Public Health, Part 3 of the Register. They have also issued the *Standards of Proficiency for Specialist Community Public Health Nurses*,[10] and these standards are grouped into four domains:

- search for health needs
- stimulation of awareness of health needs

- influence of policies affecting health
- facilitating health-enhancing activities

These four domains are subdivided into principles, so that any training for specialist nurse practitioner status in occupational health will cover the ten principles of:

- Developing quality and risk management within an evaluative culture.
- Policy and strategy development and implementation to improve health and well-being.
- Promoting and protecting the working population's health and well-being.
- Surveillance and assessment of the working population's health and well-being.
- Collaborative working for health and well-being.
- Working to improve health and well-being.
- Developing health programmes and services and reducing inequalities.
- Research and development.
- Strategic leadership for health and well-being.
- Ethically managing self, people and resources to improve health and well-being.

If specialist courses are designed to cover these broad principles then they fit well into the key functions of an occupational health service. Certain clinical skills that may be required in specific areas, such as spirometry for lung function testing, or venepuncture (taking blood) for laboratory analysis, can be undertaken by trained technicians and do not require a specialist nurse. If an occupational health nurse wishes to undertake one of these procedures she would need to acquire training in that particular area. The full scope of the occupational health nurse can be found in the RCN Competencies – an integrated career and competency framework for occupational health nursing.[11]

Occupational hygienists

Occupational hygiene is about recognising, evaluating and controlling health hazards arising from work, so it works very much at the level of the premises, plant and processes. Courses leading to qualifications suitable for entry to the British Occupational Hygiene Society (BOHS) are available at a number of places around the country and start at certificate or diploma level, with some universities offering first and higher degrees. Only very large organisations or those with specific hazards and risk would employ an occupational hygienist full time, so many consultancies exist for employers to call on their expertise as and when needed. BOHS holds a Directory of Occupational Hygiene Consultants,[12] and lists consultancies able to provide qualified and experienced occupational hygienists and specialist occupational hygiene support services, with coverage throughout the UK.

Ergonomists

Ergonomics is the application of scientific information concerning humans to the design of objects, systems and environment for human use. Ergonomics comes into everything that involves people. Work systems, sports and leisure, and health and safety should all embody ergonomics principles if well designed.

Ergonomics courses usually start by building a basic knowledge of fundamental topics essential to a proper understanding of the subject. These will include psychology, anatomy and physiology, work organisation and industrial sociology, statistics and applied mathematics, design and evaluation methods and information technology. First and higher degrees are available at a number of universities around the country. There are different levels of qualification, from student and graduate through to fellow and honorary fellow. Again, only large organisations with specific hazards and risk would usually employ an ergonomist full time, so consultancies exist for employers to call on their expertise when needed. The Ergonomics Society holds a list of registered consultancies.[13]

Health and safety personnel

Health and safety personnel are usually people specifically trained in the field of health and safety. Not all people who are designated as 'safety officers' or 'safety managers' necessarily have appropriate qualifications in this field, and may be in that position by virtue of technical knowledge and experience of a particular process or substance. Those who are qualified will have undertaken a course approved by the National Examination Board in Occupational Safety and Health (NEBOSH). These are at certificate or diploma level. However, many universities offer health and safety first and higher degrees, which incorporate the certificate or diploma. The Institute of Occupational Safety and Health is the governing body and recently received Royal Charter status.[14] Again, there are different levels of chartered membership, from technician through to fellow.

Like occupational hygienists, health and safety personnel's main role is about recognising, evaluating and controlling health hazards arising from work, and works very much at the level of the premises, plant and processes, advising management about suitable control measures and accident prevention – a risk management approach.

Physiotherapists

Physiotherapists are sometimes employed by companies to advise on the musculoskeletal aspects of work processes, to help prevent musculoskeletal problems and to provide early treatment of any conditions arising from either work or leisure activities (such as sports injuries). This often means that employees can return to work early, or remain at work while receiving treatment. Large organisations may employ a physiotherapist full time but many work on a part-time or consultancy referral basis. Physiotherapy is one of the 13 health care professions governed by the Health Professions Council (HPC) and training is governed by the Chartered Society of Physiotherapists.[15]

Occupational psychologists

Occupational psychology is concerned with the performance of people at work or in training, how organisations function, and how individuals and groups behave at work. The aim in the workplace is often to increase the effectiveness of the organisation, and to improve the job satisfaction of the individual and the team. It touches other occupational areas such as ergonomics. The work can be in advisory, teaching and research roles, and to a lesser extent in technical and administrative roles.

Occupational psychologists often work for large companies and for private consultancies providing services to smaller organisations. They often work alongside other occupational health professionals and human resources. There is no requirement for psychology graduates to register with The British Psychological Society but they cannot claim chartered status unless they are so registered. Further training to obtain chartered status as an occupational psychologist is possible.

As can be seen, there is then considerable knowledge and skill available to advise employers, workers, human resources and managers on the health and safety aspects of the working environment and work systems. The type of occupational health provision will depend on the organisation, whether it is a service or manufacturing industry, the location of workers, the size of the workforce and the hazards to which they are exposed.

Types of occupational health services

From the inception of the occupational health function, doctors and nurses were employed mainly by large companies, such as the factories of the chocolate makers Fry and Cadbury, and other manufacturers such as Reckitt (cleaning products) and Clark's Shoes. Still today, it is often only the larger organisations that can afford, and therefore demonstrate the cost effectiveness of providing access to occupational health services for the workforce. However, today the different types of occupational health services are as diverse as the occupations they are set up to cover. The advent of computerisation has meant a decrease in the manual work undertaken by 'man power' and an increase in service industries. These are regarded as less hazardous occupations, but as time goes on they have subsequently been seen to have developed a whole new area of work-related health problems, many of which are stress or musculoskeletal related (see Chapter 5).

The different models of occupational health provision can be broadly divided into in-house or outsourced.

In-house occupational health

This type of occupational health service can range from a service with the full range of specialist and qualified occupational health professionals, generally employed by a larger organisation, to a much more modest service provided by perhaps one occupational health nurse supported by medical advice from a local GP, in smaller organisations. The range of services that are offered will depend not only on the hazards to which the workforce are exposed, but also on the experience and qualifications of the occupational health professionals employed and their remit.

Some occupational health services provide a primary health care facility, such as first aid, immunisations, dental care or podiatry. Occupational physicians and nurses are in a position to undertake an audit and assess the type of occupational health service that might be required by an organisation. Some organisations take advantage of this expertise to advise on the service provision that best suits their needs. Occasionally management decide to employ a doctor or nurse without fully considering the implication of what that professional person has to offer and what the limitations are of their role as governed by confidentiality and professional ethics. A lack of knowledge of the role and remit of occupational health professionals can lead to misunderstandings. This can even result in disciplinary procedures, and other employment tribunal cases such as in 'whistle-blowing' situations.

Occupational health providers

There has been a steady increase in recent years of the number of companies and consultancies offering occupational health services, especially to small and medium-sized enterprises (SMEs). Today 44% of occupational health is provided by this type of service, according to the CBI 2004 survey. The advantage of these organisations is that they offer the full range of occupational health services as and when required. What can be a down side is that, in order to cut costs, only a limited number of services are 'bought' on a contract, and the advice of the providers is not always heeded as to what the contract provision needs to cover.

What services can occupational health offer?

Cooperation and communication

Occupational health professionals can work with human resources, management and employee representatives to develop suitable policies and procedures, in line with health and safety and employment legislation and based on the best available evidence. This fulfils numbers 3, 5, 7, 8 and 11 of the functions of an occupational health service as outlined in the list on page 80.

Policies on such things as manual handling, mental health and stress, sickness absence, drug and alcohol abuse, etc. can all benefit from input and advice from the occupational health team. Involvement with the development of policies and procedures will ensure that occupational health plays a full role, and that the company and its representatives understand exactly what occupational health has to offer and the limitations imposed by confidentiality and professional ethics. Occupational health can provide professional advice on health and safety committees and help to analyse health, safety and accident statistics.

Keeping records and writing reports is a key requirement of a skilled and safe practitioner. The NMC Guidelines state that record keeping is an integral part of nursing and midwifery practice.[16] It is a tool of professional practice and not separate from the clinical care process.

The General Medical Council *Standards for Practice* say that doctors should keep clear, accurate, legible and contemporaneous patient records, including decisions made on drugs and other treatment.[17] Records and record keeping are explored in depth in Chapter 2. Occupational health doctors and nurses can also work in cooperation with local health and employment services, health centres and GPs for the benefit of the company and the workforce.

Risk assessment

Although the requirement to undertake risk assessments is placed firmly on the shoulders of the employer by the Health and Safety Executive, occupational health services can support management by undertaking their own risk assessments in order to identify the health risks in the workplace and give suitable advice to management, employees and their representatives. It is a first function of an occupational health service as well as fulfilment of functions 2, 3, 4 and 5 in the list on page 80. Without a clear knowledge of the workplace and what the work processes entail, sound advice can be compromised, and this is where occupational health can demonstrate its worth. Being 'fit for work' is not a clear-cut, yes-or-no decision; it will depend on what the worker's job entails. For example, there is a big difference between sitting at a desk on, say, reception duties and sitting in the cab of a train or heavy goods vehicle. The differences in the jobs of workers will be reflected in diverse health-related risk factors.

Whether the workplace is a healthy and safe place in which to work can be assessed initially by managers, with support and advice from health and safety officers and occupational health nurses and doctors. But specialist areas, such as chemical or substance handling, will benefit from the expertise of an occupational hygienist who can measure and monitor the environment and individual exposure to substances. Workstation and work equipment design, and planning and organisation of work, can benefit from the expertise of an ergonomist who can advise on modifications and adaptations where necessary.

Where breakdowns in health and safety occur, these may result in accidents or exposure to occupational disease. Occupational health has a duty to keep records of any people they may have treated as a result of an accident or injury at work, or in any other circumstances where treatment has been given by them. Management is required to keep accurate absence and accident records, as detailed in Chapter 2.

Health promotion, protection and surveillance

Surveillance is a broad term and encompasses a considerable amount of work undertaken by the occupational health doctors and nurses. It is not limited to their function only, however, because other members of the team play an important part, especially with regard to the surveillance of work environment factors. This topic is covered in depth in Chapter 3. List points 2 and 6 (page 80) cover these functions of an occupational health service. Health promotion incorporates all measures deliberately designed to promote health and handle disease, according to Tonnes;[18] and this is at the heart of the occupational health function.

Health promotion is also often seen as educating people about a healthy lifestyle – for example, no smoking, healthy eating, cutting down on alcohol consumption and taking more exercise – and this, too, is a key part of helping to achieve a healthy and happy workforce. Such initiatives are best pursued in conjunction with national and local health-promoting measures, but a prime function of occupational health is to look at how the work impacts on health, and health on work. As such, it should support, rather than duplicate, health-promotion initiatives offered elsewhere. The government document *Health, Work and Well-being – Caring for our Future* (Department for Work and Pensions, 2005) outlines the national strategy for the health and well-being of working age people and recognises the important role that occupational health services can play in both the public and private sectors through a variety of different models delivering work-focused support.

Mental health services

'It is not easy to define satisfactorily what is meant by mental health or positive mental health well being,' states Brennan,[19] a respected expert in the mental health field. He also says that there is, however, a consensus of agreement that people who would describe themselves as being happy possess all, or at least most, of the following characteristics: a high sense of subjective well-being, resilience, a healthy sense of humour, and good self awareness.[20] One of the most common causes of poor mental health is stress related.[21] The HSE defines stress as 'the adverse reaction people have to excessive pressure or other types of demand placed on them'.[22] Because of the high incidence and costs of stress-related illness today, the Health and Safety Executive has put in place guidance standards (see Chapter 5), which employers can aim to achieve in order to prevent stress-related ill health. As with all health and safety issues, managing stress starts with undertaking a risk assessment in the workplace of the six HSE-identified key areas (also covered in Chapter 5). Occupational health can help, guide and support employers and managers with risk assessment and stress management standards. They can also help to set up stress management initiatives, employee assistance programmes and counselling services. As stressed employees are often worried that they may be seen as weak and their condition frowned upon by their managers, doctors and nurses can provide a safe, confidential service for employees to refer to with their concerns.

Sickness, absence and rehabilitation

It is not the role of occupational health to replace the facilities provided by the NHS, such as GP services and accident and emergency services. A first aid provision is sometimes necessary on site, however. The type and size of the provision will be determined by the size and location of the workforce, as detailed in Chapter 1. There may also be instances when there is a need to risk assess the requirement for such a provision in relation to the workplace and the availability of NHS services near to it. First aid at work training has been under review for several years, following a research project published in 2003.[23] The HSE positions statement of October 2005 recommends training at two levels: six-hour emergency first aid training, requiring re-qualification every 12 months; and an 18-hour first aid at work course, requiring re-qualification every three years, but which also includes emergency first aid requiring annual re-qualification. The HSE will shortly publish a guide to carrying out first aid needs assessment for employers.

With the advent of automated external defibrillators (AEDs), occupational health services are now often asked to provide training in the use of this equipment in emergencies. It is wise to follow the latest advice from the Resuscitation Council UK (www.resus.org.uk) on who should undertake this training and the frequency of retraining.

Other aspects of absence management, in particular, sickness absence, rehabilitation and the role of occupational health will be explored in depth in Chapter 5.

Employment law perspectives

In Chapter 3 we outlined the crucially important health surveillance duty that rests with the employer and management. Where there is an occupational health service available, those professionals will play a key role in supporting the management task and providing valued services to both the employer and the employee.

The importance of the occupational health task begins from the moment the recruitment process is contemplated, as covered in Chapter 1. This applies to firms of all sizes, and whether or not there is a professional occupational health service available, or whether its functions are instead in the hands of general management or human resources.

During the cycle of employment, once an employee is in post at whatever level in an organisation, there are health and safety considerations that must be managed throughout. We have already summarised some of the key obligations in relation to health and safety at work legislation. These apply to all individuals and to all employers, whether or not there is a known injury or illness factor to consider. In Chapter 5 we look at sickness and absence specifically, together with the Disability Discrimination Act's implications, but there are many other health-related issues for employers to manage in respect of the occupational health of staff. These do not necessarily involve sickness absence but they cover a range of health-related issues that occur during the cycle of employment.

Many of the issues can affect work performance, staff turnover, morale and other key factors that contribute to business success and a committed workforce. Addressing these matters at the earliest stage can help to nip problems in the bud by tackling them positively and before they become a health, performance, conduct or legal problem.

The occupational health personnel are generally among the most trusted professionals in an organisation because of their codes of ethical and professional conduct, their advisory capacity and the impartiality they can offer to all parties. Human resources professionals who are chartered members of the Chartered Institute of Personnel and Development (CIPD) are also obliged to follow a code of conduct: the website provides details of the code for its members (www.cipd.co.uk). Occupational health and human resources can play a key part in a cohesive team approach to addressing workplace initiatives that look for early signs of problems and for examples of good working practices that can guide others to follow. Being aware of the employment rights of people at work can help in the assessment of trends and action plans for multidisciplinary teams and specialist groups to work upon to provide measurable results.

National trends can be examined to ascertain how to measure and compare these locally and internally. For example, looking at employment litigation and internal procedures for dealing with discipline, grievance and appeal processes in that way could help to address good practice ideas and identify any problem trends. The information could provide a sound basis for a training needs analysis, and perhaps give clues as to absence levels and performance trends – good or not so good.

Discrimination and unfair employment practices

The employment relationship is beset with legislation and potential litigation for the whole of its duration. The claim that the UK is an increasingly litigious society is borne out by the latest statistics derived from ACAS.[24] These show that there was again a general rise in the number of applications (ET1s) to the employment tribunals in the year ending March 2004. The types of claim, determined by the nature of the jurisdiction of the claim itself, cover the following categories; the percentages relate to the overall number of claims lodged during this period and are compared with the previous two years' percentages:

- Unfair dismissal – 39% [downward trend: compared to 44% and 47%].
- Unlawful deductions from wages – 20% [downward trend: compared to 22% and 21%].
- Breach of contract – 8% [downward trend: compared to 10% and 9%].
- Redundancy pay – 4% [upward trend: compared to 5% and 5%].
- Sex discrimination – 10% [upward trend: compared to 5% and 5%].
- Race discrimination – 3% [stable trend: compared to 3% and 3%].
- Disability discrimination – 3% [upward trend: compared to 3% and 2%].
- Working time – 2% [stable trend: compared to 2% and 2%].
- Equal pay – 2% [stable trend: compared to 2% and 2%].
- National minimum wage – 0.2% [stable trend: compared to 0.2% and 0.3%].
- Flexible working – 0.1% [new category].
- Other – 8% [upward trend: compared to 4% and 3%].

There is a rise, then, in discrimination cases evidenced by the sex and disability discrimination statistics. The category 'Other' may include other discrimination claims such as those relating to religion or belief, sexual orientation, etc.

The levels of tribunal awards for different types of cases are also relevant for employers to consider. The basic awards and compensation levels in unfair dismissal cases have prescribed methods of calculation, which include a ceiling of the number of weeks that can be counted, and the maximum level of a week's pay within that calculation for tribunals to use in their awards as follows.

As from 1 February 2006, the figures for unfair dismissal claims as above are (previous figures in brackets):

- One week's pay: £290 [£280].
- Maximum compensatory award: £58,400 [£56,800].
- Minimum basic award for defined dismissals (trade union, health and safety, etc.): £4000 [£3800].

These levels are reviewed in February each year. They apply to dismissal cases, and similar calculations currently apply to statutory redundancy pay. In addition to the basic awards, eligible employees who are found to have been unfairly dismissed can also receive other payments including, for example, an award for the manner of dismissal, loss of future earnings and other items that count as remuneration, such as pensions.

Awards for discrimination are not capped, and those compensatory awards, while following some guidelines for calculation, are not limited. In many instances aggrieved employees may make tribunal applications covering more than one category of allegation: for example, unfair dismissal and discrimination on the grounds of disability.

Since 1 October 2004, employers and employees have been obliged to follow the Employment Act 2002 (Dispute Resolution) Regulations 2004,[25] which introduced a minimum legal standard that must be observed by all employers in dismissal, disciplinary and grievance proceedings, as mentioned previously.

A further extension of civil rights was introduced at the end of 2005 with the new Civil Partnership Act 2004. This has created a new legal relationship of civil partnership, which two people of the same sex can form by signing a registration document. Discrimination law now covers civil partners. Employers will therefore need to adapt workplace policies so as to ensure that civil partnership is recognised in the same way as marriage in pension schemes, staff benefits, next of kin contact details, parental leave rights, etc.

Travelling abroad

Many jobs involve some foreign travel today. There are occupations that entail travel as an everyday and intrinsic part of the job, such as air or shipping crew, and others that require regular travel in order for the employee to carry out essential duties that are not transport related. There are other situations where an employee is posted abroad for a period. All of these situations have potential health-related considerations.

If the starting and return point is the UK, and if the contract of employment and currency of salary is UK based, then there will usually be a basis to preserve UK employment rights. But where overseas postings are a factor, or where duties are centred abroad, there can be circumstances in which employees may not have the same rights as those who are home based. The law and its application are complex and each case will turn on its particular facts, so these parameters are a very general guide only. It is also important to note that, employment rights aside, other countries will have different laws and different standards of behaviour that are expected both at work and in general. Occupational health information, risk assessment and research are essential to good employment practice in protecting the health and well-being of employees working abroad.

The contract of employment sets out the terms that are applicable to the job the person is employed to do. If a contract provides for a substantial move, or goes further to include posting abroad, the employee will usually be expected to comply when the move comes up as long as the employer deals with the move reasonably. Even when there is no clause in the contract referring to a move, if there is a sound business reason for the employer requiring it the courts might well expect the employee to cooperate, provided the employer consults with him properly. Where it was fairly predictable that a move would be required, a resignation prompted by the move might not necessarily be found to be constructive dismissal. A fairly obvious example would be the situation where the company has offices in several countries; at interview the employee is told that travel might be involved and is enthusiastic about the prospect, and the employee is aware that foreign postings are expected. A court could find that there is an implied term in the contract of employment that, to ensure business efficacy, staff are prepared to work abroad.

The existing contract may have an explicit 'mobility clause'. This provides for reasonable changes in the employment contract, including a change of the site where the employee is required to work. One such change, particularly if the company is multinational or has offices abroad, would be that the employee is to be stationed abroad. However, change must be implemented reasonably so as to give the employee enough time to deal with the domestic and other changes ancillary to a move.

An opportunity may arise for the employee to work abroad. If there is no provision in the contract for a change but the employee could be persuaded by the right terms, those can be negotiated. Terms should be negotiated carefully so as to cover matters such as health care insurance, moving costs, accommodation, reporting structure, etc. Where the terms are not satisfactory to the employee, he has the right to refuse to go. Any attempt to impose the change could amount to a breach of contract.

Good employment practice takes account of the fact that employees also have duties and obligations outside work: their own health and personal circumstances, children's schools, their partner's or a dependent relative's needs.

Employment protection rights are restricted to the UK. This means that people who work abroad may also not be protected by UK health and safety legislation and, save for acts of harassment or acts of discrimination taking place within Great Britain, they may be dependent on local legislation.

In law, the Employment Rights Act 1996 makes it clear that:

(1) an employer must give an employee a statement of initial employment particulars
(2) ... within two months of the start of employment
(3) and (4) details relating to pay, pensions, holidays, job title and description and length of fixed term contract.

For employees who might be sent to work abroad, section 1(4)(k) is important. This requires particulars to be given:

> where the employee is required to work outside the UK for a period of more than one month – covering
>
> (i)   the period for which he is to work outside the UK;
>
> (ii)   the currency in which remuneration is to be paid while he is working outside the UK;
>
> (iii) any additional remuneration payable to him, and any benefits to be provided to or in respect of him, by reason of his being transferred to work outside the UK, and
>
> (iv) any terms and conditions relating to his return to the UK.

Workers' health and safety rights are confirmed by a raft of legislation derived from Europe, to ensure that they work safe hours in safe places using safe systems of work. Where health and safety legislation is breached, the Health and Safety Executive exists to bring redress to bear on the errant employer. In addition, the employee has recourse to litigation in the courts and tribunals to achieve recompense for any harm suffered.

Discrimination can sometimes have an adverse effect on the health of victims. UK law has a very wide remit to ensure equality of treatment and opportunity in the workplace. Going to work abroad may mean giving up some of that protection. The risk of loss of employment protection may have to be weighed against the benefits of a foreign job, whether it is an independent venture or an employment posting abroad. The employer must take all reasonable steps to ensure that the transferred employee is going to work in a safe place, even if the employee is being seconded to another employer.

Although the duty on the main employer cannot be delegated, the courts consider all the factors relating to the new location, the nature of the premises where the work is to be done and the experience of the employee in doing the work that he has been sent to do. Above all, the courts will be concerned with the amount of control the UK employer can exert practically or at all at the distant location.

Employers should ascertain the risks of working on the site to which the employee is being sent in a process similar to the domestic risk assessment required under the Management of Health and Safety at Work Regulations 1999.

It is important for the employee to understand the terms and conditions relating to his employment, and to know how to deal with problems and what sources of help will be available to him. It will also be useful if, for example, an employee is to be seconded abroad for a period that he is told what the position will be with the job he left behind upon his return.

The courts have recognised that a temporary posting overseas will not necessarily deprive the employee of the protection of the Employment Rights Act 1996, insofar as dismissals are concerned. However, other protections of the Employment Rights Act may not be available to employees working abroad. These include matters that are almost taken for granted here, such as health and safety, whistle-blowing and wage protection.

Countries in the European Union have supposedly similar legislation to the UK, but there are differences within each member state. The EU Posted Workers' Directive No. 96/71 sets out standards to be applied to workers who 'for a limited period' carry out their work on a transfer to another EU state. These ensure that the basic health and safety protection is in place, including working time restraints and equal treatment. Nonetheless, within Europe differences in other states' employment legislation should be checked. Outside Europe, this is absolutely essential.

Case law

In *United Bank Ltd* v. *Akhtar* [1989] IRLR 507, the Employment Appeal Tribunal held that mobility clauses should be implemented fairly. There is an implied term that, when an employee is required to move, in accordance with an agreed term in his contract, he will be dealt with so as to maintain trust and confidence in his employer. The Bank gave Mr Akhtar a few days' notice that he would be moving from headquarters in Leeds to a branch office in Birmingham. His contract provided for the move, but the court said that he should have been given reasonable notice of any proposed transfer. Further, the employer did not fulfil its contractual obligation to provide relocation expenses.

In *Square D Ltd* v. *Cook* [1992] IRLR 34, the Court of Appeal considered whether there was any negligence by the employer who sent its employee to work in the Middle East. He fell into an uncovered hole on a construction site that he was visiting as a surveyor. He was injured, and sued his employer in negligence. It was held that the employer's duty was generally met by inspecting the site and ensuring that the occupiers were reasonable and competent to ensure its safety. This employer had done what it reasonably could to ensure safety, given the great distance involved. From this decision, it appears that there is no absolute duty to take reasonable steps to ensure the health and safety of an employee posted abroad, although it is good practice to do so. Reasonable steps would be to ascertain the work that is to be done and how it is done, and inspect the premises where it will be carried out and determine whether or not they are defective. If staff are sent to work abroad for a longish period, an employer might be expected to visit the site personally, inspect it and ensure that local management and personnel know of and understand health and safety obligations. It would be reasonable and recommended best practice to explain any risks to the travelling employee so that he or she can be provided with suitable training or equipment to cope with problems. It should be borne in mind that health and safety issues can change rapidly, and a site that is safe one day can be dangerous on another.

The employee should ascertain what insurance cover is to be provided, if any, and for what purposes. The Court of appeal in *Reid* v. *Rush & Tomkins Group plc* [1989] IRLR 265 held that an employer is not under a duty to insure an employee seconded abroad against special risks, nor is there a duty on the employer to advise the employee to take out the requisite insurance cover. It is, nevertheless, good practice for the employer to do so. Mr Reid was injured in a car accident while working abroad. The driver was not insured and Mr Reid then learned that his employer had not insured him against the risk of accidents. On the judgment of the Court of Appeal, the employer was not negligent in failing to warn Mr Reid that he would be uninsured while working abroad. There is a need for prudence on both sides of the employee relationship: the employer to insure as he chooses, and the employee to check what cover is being provided.

Stress, bullying and harassment

The psychological health and safety of employees is just as important in law as their physical well-being. Stress, bullying and other forms of harassment, cruelty or violence that could affect the mental health of the employee should be rated as of equal importance to physical health risk factors. These essential assessments will reduce the risk of litigation only if action is taken to correct defects and there is evidence of this. Seeking out causal factors, assessing risk and addressing problems are key occupational health functions. Long before an illness develops, there may be trends and signs that can be picked up so that matters are able to be addressed before they become problems. Health and safety inspections, health surveillance and staff turnover are all exercises that can highlight areas that may warrant further investigations.

Elements of causation of stress-related illness

We will look in more detail at stress-related illness in Chapter 5, but for the purpose of this section we must also consider that bullying in all its forms can give rise to damaging stress upon the victim. Any illness must be shown to have been caused by the employer's act or omission in order for there to be a basis for a claim for damages. But before damage to health does take place, setting standards of workplace conduct and monitoring working practice can help to address problems at the outset. Stress can be both positive and negative. When it switches from one to the other then motivation and productivity go down. The morale of the individual and sometimes that of the whole team can sink too.

The TUC has highlighted the following issues as being considered the main causes of negative stress at work:[26]

- Workload – 74%.
- Cuts in staff – 53%.
- Change at work – 44%.
- Long hours – 39%.
- Shift work – 30%.
- Bullying – 30%.
- Other factors – inadequate training/supervision, poor and/or dangerous working conditions, poor relationships with colleagues.

Bullying and discrimination

Physical and verbal abuse and harassment may (depending on, for example, the gender, sexual orientation, race, religion, disability, and – from October 2006 – age of the affected person) be prohibited discriminatory behaviour under the various anti-discrimination laws now in force. Bullying is often a manifestation of discrimination, and can be physical or verbal or both. Sometimes it does not result in obvious health problems or absenteeism, but it is always cruel to the individual and thus must impact on their work.

Complaints of discrimination do not require any length of service to entitle the employment tribunal to have jurisdiction to allow the claim. If the working environment is intolerable, but not for discriminatory reasons, then one year's service is required to bring a claim for constructive dismissal.

The Health and Safety Executive gives guidance for coping with and preventing work-related violence. Whereas its 1986 definition of violence referred only to assaults by members of the public, the 1996 definition is 'any incident in which an employee is abused, threatened or assaulted in circumstances relating to their work',[27] implicitly including workplace bullying. Bullying behaviour includes non-verbal insults, such as excluding colleagues from communal activities within or outside the workplace: the equivalent of 'sending someone to Coventry'. Verbal bullying covers the spectrum of insults, threats and oppressive management style. Bullying may also extend to the arena of actual or threatened physical violence. Various forms of bullying are covered by different areas of the law: violence or the threat thereof constitutes an assault, which is a criminal offence. Where the behaviour affects the health and safety of the victim, criminal aspects of health and safety law are invoked.

Unacceptable behaviour in the workplace can and should result in disciplinary procedures that are governed by aspects of employment law. A victim who is damaged physically or psychologically has recourse to the civil law in which damages are recoverable under different torts (civil wrongs). These are:

- Negligence on the part of the employer, who is vicariously liable for the acts of his bullying employee.
- Intimidation or harassment, whether by the employer directly or a bullying employee.
- Assault which is both a criminal offence and a civil wrong.
- Under criminal law further protection to victims is provided by the Protection from Harassment Act 1997.

Employer checklist: bullying and discrimination

Procedural steps it is necessary to show as having been taken if bullying or other forms of harassment are indicated will include the following:

- A thorough investigation.
- A written statement from the person making the allegations.
- An invitation to the person making the allegations to commence proceedings.
- An explanation of procedure, including the information that confidentiality may not be completely guaranteed, as natural justice demands that the alleged harasser be informed of the nature of the accusations against him or her, and that the interests of potential further victims be protected.
- Disciplinary procedures should follow, particularly where the harasser continues the offensive behaviour.

Vicarious liability

In addition to the responsibility of the perpetrator of the act(s) of discrimination, anti-discrimination legislation provides that the employer will be liable for the acts or omissions of managers and employees unless they have done everything that is 'reasonably practicable' to prevent any such discrimination. It will usually be necessary to show that that a proper policy has been introduced, that staff have been trained in it, and that it is monitored and reviewed for effectiveness – a key part of the 'reasonably practicable steps'. Thus, the employer will need to show:

- That he did all in his power to prevent sexual, racial, age, gender, religious or disability harassment, usually by way of a written policy that is brought to the attention of all staff.
- That any complaint was brought to his attention.
- That timely and appropriate action was taken.

An employer cannot simply rely on the existence of written policies. The policy must be pursued with necessary actions. An employer with no written policy on harassment as a disciplinary offence and related procedures is likely to find it difficult to prove a valid defence to a charge that entails joint responsibility with the perpetrator of the offence, unless the acts that were carried out were clearly beyond the bounds of work.

As a general guide to monitoring standards, the following key points may be useful:

- Written polices and procedures – train, review, monitor, revise, communicate.
- Identify workplace standards of conduct, performance and culture.
- Conduct risk assessments.
- Create an environment of trust and confidence in the occupational health service – ensure that staff feel safe in bringing attention to their own health concerns, workplace health and safety matters, 'whistle-blowing', bullying, etc.
- Have a policy that allows staff to have complaints or concerns (discrimination, harassment, bullying, stress) investigated properly and sensitively.
- Have a policy that allows employees to be fairly protected from malicious or unfounded allegations.
- Train and communicate policies and procedures comprehensively. Resistance to change can be overcome through good standards of communication and education.
- Keep good records.
- Ensure that fast and clear investigations take place. Consider the benefits of a clear and unequivocal apology coupled with a remedial action plan.
- Have the right systems and people in place to avoid repetition of problems and complaints.

If prevention fails and a member of staff is injured in a violent incident, the consequences may be both physical and psychological. Minor physical aspects usually heal well, but residual long-term psychological problems present a risk. The occupational health team are often trained to debrief the victims of all levels of incident, and thereafter to use counselling or refer them on to an appropriate counsellor where necessary. Where other employees have observed the incident(s), particularly where there has been bullying or other psychological trauma, those employees should be seen so that their needs may be assessed. Employees should be informed – without divulging confidentiality – of certain facts concerning an incident if this is relevant to the prevention of gossip and rumours that may magnify or inflame the situation, with follow-up as to the outcome and the reasons for any management decision. The proper treatment for bullying is bringing redress upon the bully and providing support for the victim together with others who may have been indirectly affected.

Employer checklist: vicarious liability

Effective steps that an employer should have taken to avoid being jointly or separately liable for the acts of employees include:

- A fully publicised equal opportunities/treatment policy.
- An active training programme in equal treatment and equal opportunities.
- A disciplinary code itemising 'serious or persistent acts of harassment' as gross misconduct.
- Protection from victimisation where complaints have been made, regardless of whether the complaint is upheld.
- A proper grievance and appeal procedure to handle all types of complaints.
- Fair, appropriate and supportive facilities available to victims.
- Information as to warnings or other disciplinary outcomes so as to ensure that persons who have committed previous acts of harassment are known and any further acts are dealt with promptly.

Case law: working conditions

Unpleasant working conditions take their toll of the health of employees, both directly and indirectly. The case of *Walker* v. *Northumberland County Council* [1995] IRLR was a warning to employers to take care of the psychological health of their staff. Mr Walker, a social worker, suffered a nervous breakdown as a result of the stressful nature of his work. His employers undertook to ensure that he would not be required to undertake the same sort of stressful caseload upon his return to work after illness, but he rapidly became overworked and subject to stress. He then suffered a second nervous breakdown for which his employers were held liable because by then it was reasonably foreseeable that he would become ill unless he worked within safe parameters that took account of his fragile health.

Stress-related illness is likely to affect vulnerable persons, and employers must be aware that too much stress or working under threat of violence, whether by bullying, or harassment, or other means, may lead to illness unless appropriate steps are taken. Mr Walker's case carries a clear message to employers that they must take reasonably practicable steps to reduce stress that could otherwise lead to illness. As in all other work-related illness, the affected employee who seeks compensation will need to show a medical diagnosis and expert opinion that their specific condition was caused or exacerbated by work and that the employer knew or ought to have known that working conditions could and should have been remedied.

Case law: workplace discrimination

A single incident of adverse treatment can be sufficient to amount to bullying, which may also be an act of discrimination. In *Bracebridge Engineering Ltd* v. *Darby* [1992] IRLR3, EAT, Ms Darby suffered an incident of sexual harassment and assault by two male colleagues. They were not disciplined and so she resigned, complaining of constructive dismissal and sex discrimination. Both complaints were upheld by the Employment Appeal Tribunal: a single act of sexual harassment was a 'detriment' under the Sex Discrimination Act 1975 (SDA). The facts of the case were that two male supervisors were annoyed by Ms Darby's continually leaving work early. One evening they accosted her as she was leaving work; they took her into a room, made a series of lewd remarks and committed a sexual assault. The employer was found to have been vicariously liable for the acts of the supervisors who were carrying out their authorised duty (time-keeping) in a completely improper way.

The employer is responsible if the acts were carried out during the course of and in connection with the discriminator's work. It was held in *Porcelli* v. *Strathclyde Regional Council* [1986] ICR 564 that sexual harassment falls within the scope of the SDA as it is part of the mischief that the Act sets out to contain. Mrs Porcelli was subjected to unacceptable, vindictive behaviour by her male colleagues who were attempting to make life so unpleasant for her that she would seek a job transfer. They made lewd and suggestive remarks and brushed their bodies against her. That treatment would not have been meted out to an equally disliked man and was therefore held to be direct discrimination.

In *Jones* v. *Tower Boot Company Limited* [1997] 2 All ER 406, the case established that the employer could also be held to be vicariously liable for the acts of employees who were not acting in the course of their work. Employees insulted a black colleague, generally taunted him and even branded him with hot metal. The Court of Appeal held that serious acts of violence carried out against an employee were broadly within the ambit of 'in the course of employment', and the employer was therefore liable for the actions of its employees.

Case law: no laughing matter

All too often so-called practical jokes go wrong and end up with someone suffering at the hands of the prankster or perpetrator. The employer who turns a blind eye to this kind of culture or who fails to realise what is taking place can be found to be liable. The case law is long established.

In *Chapman* v. *Oakleigh Animal Products Ltd* [1970] 8 KIR 1063, a group of workmen told a junior employee to put his hand up the spout of a grinding machine, with the intention of spraying ground ice through the spout as a joke. The joke went wrong, and the employee was injured. The employer was held to be liable. While the employer had not authorised the men in question to injure the young employee, it had authorised them to give him instructions. The young employee had put his hand into the grinder as a result of instructions that were clearly given in the course of the employment.

The employer's duty of care to protect the health and safety of staff applies to danger from other employees as well as from equipment and other workplace hazards. In *Hudson* v. *Ridge Manufacturing Co Ltd* [1957] 2 All ER 229 CA, an employee persistently tripped up fellow employees as a 'joke', and eventually he injured someone. The Court of Appeal held the employer liable on the basis that it knew the employee's conduct was a potential source of danger, and in those circumstances, the Court said, 'a duty lies fairly and squarely on the employer to remove the source of danger'.

Working time regulations

The Working Time Regulations 1998 have been updated since they came into force in October 1998 (see p. 100 for details of amendments). It is likely that they will go on developing, and it is recommended that regular updates on the legal position and advisory guidance be checked routinely: the website www.dti.gov.uk provides a very comprehensive information section for this purpose.

In summary only, then, the key points from an occupational health perspective cover current regulations, which at present include, but are not limited to, the following:

- Individual employees are currently still allowed to opt out of the 48-hour week limit in the UK, with employers being obliged only to keep 'up-to-date records' of all workers who have opted out.
- Workers must not be forced to work for more than 48 hours a week on average.
- There must be regular rest breaks, during work shifts and to allow daily and weekly rest.
- Special rules for young workers apply for their work rest periods, breaks and hours limitations. For example, they currently may not ordinarily work more than eight hours a day or 40 hours a week, although there are certain permitted exceptions, and there are special daily and weekly limits that should also be checked as to the up-to-date regulations.
- Every worker is entitled to annual holiday of four weeks' paid leave. This currently does not include bank holidays, but the rule should be checked for the updated position as this is under review.
- Special rules apply to night workers. Night time is defined as between 11 pm and 6 am. There are hours limitations that apply specifically to night workers when their hours of work are averaged. There are particular rules that prohibit this averaging, however, when there are special hazards identified with their work or where heavy mental or physical strain is required. The MHSW Regulations apply to risk assessment of these factors.
- Employers must offer night workers a free health assessment before they start regular night work. The health assessment must be of two parts: a questionnaire and a medical examination, where appropriate. The latter need only be necessary for the individual if there are any concerns raised by the questionnaire. Employers are advised to seek advice from a suitably qualified health professional in devising and assessing the questionnaire. The DTI website also provides a helpful sample health questionnaire that can be adapted for use.

The Working Time Regulations state that working time is when someone is 'working, at his employer's disposal and carrying out his activity or duties'. This includes:

- Working lunches, such as business lunches.
- When a worker has to travel as part of his or her work, for example a 24-hour mobile repairman or travelling salesman.
- When a worker is undertaking training that is job related.

- Time spent abroad working if a worker works for an employer who carries on business in Great Britain.

It does not include:

- Routine travel between home and work.
- Rest breaks when no work is done.
- Time spent travelling outside normal working time.
- Training such as non-job-related evening classes or day-release courses.

Certain workers are not subject to these regulations because they are governed by sector-specific provisions. These are currently:

- Sea transport, as covered by the Seafarers' Directive (1999/63/EC).
- Mobile workers in inland waterways and lake transport.
- Workers on board sea-going fishing vessels.
- Air transport, as covered by the Aviation Directive (2000/79/EC). This Directive affects all mobile workers in commercial air transport (both flight crew and cabin crew), but not workers employed in general aviation.

Others who are subject only to certain provisions of the general regulations are mobile workers in road transport, as covered by the Road Transport Directive (2002/15/EC). This Directive affects mobile workers participating in road transport activities covered by EU drivers' hours rules, including drivers, members of the vehicle crew, and any others who form part of the travelling staff.

From 1 August 2003, UK workers became subject to the Road Transport Directive benefit to paid annual leave and the right to health assessments for night workers under the general scope of the Working Time Regulations.

Also from 1 August 2003, the Working Time Regulations were extended to cover to the following sectors:

- Workers in air transport, other than those covered by the Aviation Directive.
- All workers in rail transport.
- Workers in road transport, other than those subject to the Road Transport Directive.
- Non-mobile workers in sea fishing, sea transport, inland waterways and lake transport.
- All workers in other work at sea, such as offshore work in the oil and gas industry.

Working time limits for doctors in training are being phased in gradually. From 1 August 2004, doctors in training became subject to weekly working time limits, which are being phased in as follows: 58 hours from 1 August 2004 to 31 July 2007; 56 hours from 1 August 2007 to 31 July 2009; 48 hours from 1 August 2009.

Fatigue must be considered in all risk assessments as tiredness can lead to stress, accidents and physical injury. This is a factor even if a worker has agreed to work longer hours. In addition to working time records and monitoring, proper rest breaks must be in place and job rotations should be considered where appropriate. This is particularly relevant to specific duties: for example, production lines and repetitive strain injuries risk assessment, Display Screen Equipment working, and driving jobs.

Case law

In *Hone* v. *Six Continents Retail Ltd* [2005] EWCA Civ 922, the Court held that when deciding whether psychiatric injury is reasonably foreseeable (for the purpose of a stress at work claim), it is proper for the court to take into account that the employer is breaching the maximum average 48-hour working week (and the rest provisions) contained in the Working Time Regulations 1998. Mr Hone was awarded £21,840 damages for the psychiatric injury caused by stress at his work as a licensed house manager.

In *Johnstone* v. *Bloomsbury Health Authority* [1992] QB 333 [1991], it was made clear that the employer owes a duty of care to safeguard the employee's health and safety at work. That duty is one that is implied and is an overriding one whatever the parties may agree in a contract of employment. Dr Johnstone was a junior doctor who expressly agreed to work long hours while training. His health suffered as a result. The employer argued that he had agreed to work the long hours, which were the norm for the job. But the case showed that any such contractual agreement has to be subject to health and safety being the priority. That remains the case today: even if an employee has agreed to waive the working hours limitation under the Working Time Regulations, the employer could still be liable should his health suffer as a result.

Drugs and alcohol

The employer has duties and obligations under the Health and Safety at Work etc. Act 1974 (HASWA) and subordinate legislation such as the Management of Health and Safety at Work Regulations 1999 (MHSWR). There are also obligations under other legislation including the Road Traffic Act 1988 and the Transport and Works Act 1992. These stipulate that drivers must not be under the influence of alcohol while driving. Under the Misuse of Drugs Act 1971, it is an offence for any person knowingly to permit the production, supply or use of controlled substances on their premises, except when prescribed by a doctor.

There are also industry-specific regulations covering particular sectors, such as the Railways (Safety Case) Regulations 2000 (as amended April 2003) and the Railways and Transport Safety Act 2003 – Aviation: Alcohol and Drugs, together with Aeronautical Information Circular 58/2000 *Medication, Alcohol and Flying*. Industry-specific regulations, as exampled within the transport industries mentioned, require employers and operators to use all due diligence to ensure that their workers are not unfit though alcohol, drug or other substance abuse.

The Air Navigation Order (ANO) sets out a definition for flight crew and other safety-critical personnel that can also serve as a valuable basis for most other employments in terms of making it clear how an employer regards drug and alcohol misuse at work:

'The effect of intoxication, through alcohol or drugs, on aviation personnel has significant safety implications. The ANO, which is the main aviation safety regulatory legislation reference in the UK, provides that no member of an aircraft's crew, a licensed maintenance engineer or an air traffic control officer shall be under the influence of drink or drugs to such an extent as to impair his/her capacity to so act.'

Employment policies should be in place to ensure that employees in all workplaces know what standards are expected of them and their colleagues. Many employers have comprehensive policies covering substance abuse in general. It is essential that this is the case and that there is an up to date policy for dealing with drug abuse, including solvents, as well as alcohol.

Many professionals working in occupational health and human resources will be aware that normal policies can become a particular problem when employees have something to celebrate. Alcohol, the essential ingredient in many traffic and other accidents and the common factor in many incidents of violence, is not always a source of endless good cheer. Many jobs, trades and professions exist where the effects of alcohol, even in low doses, render proper performance of duties impossible. All employers need to have a designated alcohol policy, with drinking-related offences clearly stated and subject to disciplinary action including the sanction of summary dismissal for gross misconduct.

A standard alcohol policy can be quite short and along the lines of: 'All staff are forbidden to consume alcohol while on duty, prior to going on duty, and on company premises.' Some policies are more leniently worded, and qualified by a statement prohibiting drinking 'to the extent that it would endanger safety and impair judgement'. However, problems can emerge from any allowance that does not prescribe some form of limit on when, what and how much alcohol is allowed. A comprehensive policy will cover the range of issues including what is acceptable, where, when, prohibition rules, testing, and disciplinary and treatment issues.

Although alcohol abuse is easily categorised as a disciplinary issue, the law takes account of its addictive nature and many organisations deal with alcoholics as if they suffer from a disease that requires and is capable of treatment. In order to assess the extent of any problem, it is useful to include a term in the contract of employment that allows for alcohol or drug testing in random or need-to-know situations. Tests can only be carried out with the consent of the employee but unreasonable refusal can be taken into account.

Alcoholics are recognised within law as suffering from a disease in which the craving for drink can produce an abnormality of the mind so that its use becomes involuntary. Counselling and treatment may be offered prior to instigation of disciplinary proceedings but there is often likely to be an overlap, with performance issues that could come quite properly under disciplinary sanction. Alcohol-related problems could sometimes merit a period of leave in the interests of the affected employee. Dismissal or any action short of dismissal that might be deemed necessary will not be fraught with the perils of discrimination issues, as addiction to alcohol is not a condition protected by the Disability Discrimination Act 1995.

Thus, the general safeguards for employees covering physical and mental impairment do not apply, although fair procedures should, as always, be followed. It should also be noted that conditions that arise from the causal factor of alcoholism may be covered by the DDA.

The Health and Safety Executive publish guidance entitled *Don't Mix It: A Guide For Employers on Alcohol at Work*. This is essential reading for those drafting an alcohol policy.

In addition, employers now face the challenge of handling so-called recreational drugs usage by their employees. This may range from the use of illegal drugs to the problem of prescribed drugs and their effect on the employee's work. Smoking at work may also fall into this category. The company disciplinary policy must be clear as to what the employer will regard as misconduct or gross misconduct.

In general terms, coming to work under the influence of illegal drugs is a conduct issue and may be regarded as a gross misconduct. Some employers may choose, having regard to the particular circumstances of a case, to treat the employee who is seeking treatment for an addiction of this nature in the same way as one with an alcohol-dependency illness, but this will generally be exceptional in most industries. Illegal drugs usage is against the law, whereas alcohol consumption is not.

Where the employee is believed to have any kind of drug-related problem, medical evidence will be important. Some employers require workers to agree, as a term of their contract, to screening for alcohol and drugs. Where an employee suspected of drug taking refuses to undergo such tests, his employers may make a judgement on this refusal and look to the other reasonable grounds they have to believe that drug misuse has taken place.

Where criminal offences outside work are committed relating to drugs, this can be treated as a disciplinary matter if it affects the employee's ability to do his work or breaches the contractual relationship. The matter must be investigated within the disciplinary and appeal procedures, and each case would have to be judged on its own facts and circumstances.

If the employee is suspected of having a problem related to work conduct or performance in relation to prescribed drugs, medical reports will be vital. If the drugs are required for a medical condition and no alternative treatment with lesser side effects can be offered then the Disability Discrimination Act's reasonable adjustments question may be relevant for consideration by the employer.

Smoking at work will usually be prohibited except in designated areas at designated times. Employers are not obliged to make special arrangements for any right to smoke at work or to give time off to smokers. Good practice will ensure that some provision might be made through occupational health advice to help smokers give up their habit when no-smoking policies are introduced. Ill feeling can be caused within work teams, however, if smokers are allowed to disappear at regular intervals during working time to have a cigarette. Policies should make it clear that, if unauthorised, smoking breaks are unacceptable and regarded as absence from duty without permission. It seems likely that a ban on workplace smoking will be the subject of specific legislation.

Case law: misconduct dismissals

In *Williams and Others* v. *Whitbread Beer Company Ltd* [1996] CA (IDS Brief 572), the factors considered in the judgment included contributory conduct by the employees' being drunk and disorderly, and mitigation arising from the employer's condoning the drinking that led to the misconduct. Whitbread Beer Company Ltd had organised a two-day training seminar, attended by W, T and S, at one of its hotels. On the first evening, delegates were allowed to charge their drinks to their room bills, which were paid by their employer. W, T and S all drank a large quantity of alcohol and became rowdy. One employee was abusive to a senior manager who had asked him to 'tone it down', and the other two had what could be best described as an 'eventful' evening. Eventually matters erupted into an argument that led to T throwing his beer over S, who responded by swinging a punch at T. All three employees were dismissed.

The tribunal held that although the behaviour of all three employees had been deplorable, their dismissal was outside the band of reasonable responses open to a reasonable employer. The employees' misconduct had taken place outside working hours and had to be seen in the context of a heavy drinking session that had been paid for by the employer. The case went up to the Court of Appeal, which upheld the tribunal's decision. The employees' awards were, however, reduced to take account of their own contribution, by their misconduct, to their dismissals.

Employers can require high standards of conduct and take a strict view of misconduct offences during any festivities in circumstances where there is a concern for safety or the welfare of others. In *McGrath* v. *Third Generation Nursing Homes Ltd* EAT 791/93, McGrath was a registered nurse in a nursing home and was on duty on Christmas Day. The employer's disciplinary rules listed drunkenness as an example of gross misconduct. When she arrived for work the deputy matron invited her and others who were starting or finishing their shift to join her in a celebratory drink. Later that day, however, McGrath was found to be drunk and incapable of doing her work, which involved responsibility for the care of patients. She became involved in a struggle with other employees when she attempted to resume her duties, and she appeared to be very drunk. The EAT upheld the employment tribunal's finding that her dismissal was fair.

Where employers dismiss because of off-duty drug taking, other considerations may be necessary. For example, employers may argue that their reputation has been or will be damaged by the employee's conduct, or that the conduct has undermined their trust and confidence in the employee. The EAT considered this in the case of *Focus DIY Ltd* v. *Nicholson* (1994) EAT 225/94. At an office party held in August 1993, Nicholson was the most senior member of staff present. Another member of staff later complained to a senior manager that Nicholson had been smoking cannabis at the party. The employer took statements from various employees and interviewed Nicholson, who admitted that she had smoked a controlled substance at the party. She was subsequently dismissed. The EAT held that her dismissal was fair because by smoking cannabis in front of junior colleagues at a company function Nicholson had damaged her authority as a deputy manager. Key factors in the decision turned on whether a reasonable employer might consider that the smoking of cannabis was a serious matter that would have an impact on Nicholson's ability to manage. The EAT was of the opinion that a reasonable employer could have taken this view and that dismissal was within the band of responses open to a reasonable employer.

Alcoholism and the Disability Discrimination Act

In *Power* v. *Panasonic UK* [2003] IRLR 151 EAT, the question of alcohol and illness was tested. Alcoholism is excluded from the definition of disability under the DDA. The Act specifies that an addiction to or dependency on alcohol, nicotine or any other substance (other than as a result of its being medically prescribed) is outside the protection of the DDA. But a disability caused by alcoholism can be included, such as pancreas or liver disease, provided it will have a substantial long-term effect on normal day-to-day activities. Many employers do treat alcoholism as an illness, provided the employee seeks and follows a clinical recovery programme, and provided that no disciplinary offence is committed.

Random testing for drugs case

In *O'Flynn* v. *Airlinks Airport Coach Company* (2001) EAT 10269/01, it was made clear that in order to show a dismissal on the grounds of a positive drugs test was fair a number of factors would need to be evidenced by the employer. O'Flynn was not employed as a driver but her job description did require that she might be required to park the vehicles on company property. In addition, the employer had a formal policy on drugs and alcohol that stated the potential penalties for positive test results. The contract of employment should cover random and routine drug and alcohol testing and should be consistently followed. O'Flynn was found to have been fairly dismissed despite her defence that the drug misuse had been recreational and conducted during her weekend off duty.

Family-friendly working

There is a comprehensive range of statutory provisions that support the UK provisions for 'family-friendly' employment rights. These include the Maternity and Parental Leave Regulations 1999 SI No. 3312, and subsequent amendments. The rights and regulations are regularly updated and should be checked on the government-sponsored websites: www.dti.gov.uk is a good starting point that provides links to other helpful sites. Currently there are draft proposals to:

- Extend maternity leave from six to nine months from April 2007, working towards an aimed-for 12 months' paid maternity leave.
- Support improved communications between employers and employees during leave.
- Introduce a new right for mothers to transfer some of their leave and pay to fathers.
- Extend the right to request flexible working to carers of sick and disabled relatives and parents of older children.

Workers can also make a request for a change in hours, times or work location in order to care for a child under the Employment Rights Act 1996 (ERA) and Flexible Working (Procedural Requirements) Regulations 2002. They are protected in law from suffering a detriment as a result of making such a request under the Flexible Working (Eligibility, Complaints and Remedies) Regulations 2002.

It is unlawful for employers to allow someone to return to work within two weeks of giving birth.

Also under the ERA 1996 provisions, workers are entitled to take reasonable time off to care for dependants in emergency or urgent situations, or should a dependant die. This is quite different from any compassionate leave provisions that exist as part of the terms and conditions of employment but are not part of the dependant leave provisions under ERA.

Case law

In *Foster* v. *Cartwright Black* [2004] ICR 1728 EAT, the courts clarified that the right to time off for dependant leave 'in consequence of the death of a dependant', as set out in ERA, is intended to cover leave for arranging and attending a funeral, registering a death, applying for probate and making other urgent practical arrangements; but it was not intended to be a right to paid compassionate leave. This remains a matter of employment policy choice, which it is voluntary on the part of the employer to offer to staff as a special paid leave provision.

Bereavement is handled by different people in different ways, but it can sometimes be a trigger for a change in how people react to stress or in their work performance. Positive employment policies will anticipate how these situations can be handled and give pointers to good practice options that will help and support the individual employee at a potentially difficult time. Again, the services of occupational health can play a vital role in such situations: counselling can be useful to some people, risk assessment can show whether a temporary change in hours or duties might prevent an accident or illness from developing, and of course the trusted 'shoulder to lean on' can be extremely supportive at these times.

There is no obligation on employers to pay the employee while he is on this kind of leave but many do so in certain cases. Some employers choose to allow compassionate leave with pay to cover bereavement absence, for a limited time. There is much to be said for doing so, as provisions that allow some necessary time off, with or without pay, can stop people going on sick leave in those situations simply because there are no other means by which they can take time off.

Case law

Qua v. *John Ford Morrison Solicitors* [2003] IRLR 184 EAT provides an example as to how the courts can deal with the right to time off for dependants. ERA provides that it is automatically unfair to dismiss someone for exercising that statutory right.

Mrs Qua took 17 days' leave to deal with her son's medical problems during a nine-month period. Her case failed at the employment tribunal because it was found that she had failed to comply with her obligation under s.57A(2) to tell her employer 'as soon as reasonably practicable . . . how long she expected to be absent'. The Employment Appeal Tribunal sent the case back to the Employment Tribunal for it to reconsider its findings. The grounds for doing so were that the right given by legislation is to take a reasonable amount of time off work so as to deal with unexpected events affecting dependants and so as to be able to deal with an immediate crisis. Time could also be taken to make longer-term care arrangements for dependants if so required. However, the law does not create a right for employees to take time off to take general care of a child who is ill. An underlying medical condition such as asthma, involving, for example, regular relapses, does not fall within the scope of ERA's provisions. The basis of the right is to provide for time off to cope with an immediate crisis and reasonable time off to make arrangements but not for time off to care for the dependant themselves. The court also directed that a 'reasonable' amount of time off should be evaluated by a tribunal without reference to any ill-effect on the employer's business. According to the Judge, 'The operational needs of the employer cannot be relevant to a consideration of the amount of time an employee reasonably needs to deal with emergency circumstances of the kind specified . . .' Thus, although the employer has needs in relation to the running of the business, these are not relevant to the wording of the legislation, which imposes a duty on employers to permit employees to take time off work in the circumstances described without fear of reprisals, so long as they comply with legal requirement to notify the employer about the reason for absence and, unless they cannot do so before they return to work, how long they expect to be absent.

A further case that illustrated the latter point of notice to the employer was that of *MacCullough & Wallis Ltd* v. *Moore* [1992] EAT 51/02. The employee had informed her employer at the time she took dependant leave, but the EAT said that when the circumstances changed she was obliged to keep the employer informed of developments and the need for any further time off; otherwise, an employee will not have complied with due notice requirements.

Working from home

As a result of changes in working practice and the exercising of employment rights at work – for example, in matters such as flexible working and making adjustments to enable disabled people to return to work – there is now the practice of home working arrangements for most employers to consider. There is no legal definition of a 'home worker' or 'teleworker' but these workers currently make up a significant part of the UK workforce. However, these employees are covered by all health and safety legislation, and are considered to be at work in the eyes of the law when at home and on duty. Good practice suggests that when home working arrangements are made, whether for a limited time or as a more permanent arrangement, and whether for the full working week or for part of it, there should be:

- A statement of employment terms and conditions, including start, finish and break times.
- Full recognition of overtime hours and cover for absence arising from illness and annual leave
- Adequate compensation for telephone, energy, insurance and other home working costs.

- The right to communicate with other employees about work and employment relations issues, as well as measures to combat social isolation and assistance back to workplace-based employment.

Domestic legislation is already in place for home workers and this must be complied with. It includes health surveillance measures: COSHH, Health and Safety (Display Screen Equipment) Regulations, Health and Safety (Electricity at Work) Regulations, including cabling, plugs and equipment, and the Data Protection Act's requirements. Risk assessments and regular training are essential.

The Health and Safety at Work Act 1974 covers statutory protection for the health and safety of the home worker, including:

- Protection against hazards arising from work taken into the home or, for people within the household as well as the public, against hazards arising from the work.
- The duty on an employer in respect of the health and safety of employees, and 'to conduct his undertaking in such a way as to ensure . . . that persons not in his employment who may be affected thereby are not exposed to risks'.
- The duty extends to self-employed persons.
- The duty on persons supplying articles or substances for use at work, including home, exists to ensure that both are safe and without risk to health when properly used. In addition, adequate information must be provided as to the conditions of use necessary to ensure freedom from risk.

It follows that occupational health will be able to advise on:

- Ensuring that the Health and Safety at Work Policy covers home workers.
- Risk assessments being carried out, paying particular attention to home worker specifics. These may be carried out by the home workers using a checklist and should include checks on electrical equipment, work stations, etc. and other important aspects of home working such as stress, communications and employee support/supervision provisions.
- COSHH risk assessments being carried out where indicated
- Specific training for health and safety at work and in the home.
- Ensuring that adequate records are maintained for all the above.

Cars and health

Many employees drive as part of their work. Those who travel between different work locations and who visit clients using their own or a company car are regarded as being on duty when they do so. In those circumstances the employer is under a duty to ensure that they work safely when driving. This can cover a number of factors: general fitness to drive checks may be considered to be appropriate, or there may be an obligatory health surveillance requirement; licences and insurance checks should be part of company policy encompassing the requirement for employees to inform the employer of any changes to their licence; and there should be clear guidance in policies covering the unacceptability of driving while under the influence of alcohol or drugs.

In addition, from 1 December 2003 it has been a criminal offence for a person to use a hand-held mobile phone while driving a motor vehicle, whether a bus, lorry, van, car, motorcycle or other form of vehicular transport. From management's perspective, this is particularly important as there is a legal liability on an employer who causes a member of staff to use a hand-held mobile phone while driving. Although one answer to the problem of needing to be in communication with key members of staff at all times is the provision of hands-free equipment, the Highway Code (Rule 128) points out that the use of in-vehicle audio and/or visual systems can be distracting. Indeed, lack of proper control of the vehicle at all times may result in prosecution for driving without due care and attention or dangerous driving. Employers should provide guidance to employees as to proper driving standards of conduct so as to avoid direct or vicarious liability for any accidents or prosecutions arising from the use of mobile phones while driving.

Summary

Occupational health services offer employers a wide range of help, support and advice that can help to promote good health, prevent accidents and illness, save money, reduce the risk of expensive litigation and help to promote a positive workforce.

Occupational health services will be able to demonstrate to organisations that there is a sound business case to justify engaging suitably qualified occupational health professionals. Those personnel will respect the confidentiality required of their professional role, but will be able to advise and support management in their decision making and risk reduction work.

References

1. Charley, I. H. (1954) *The Birth of Industrial Nursing*. Baillière Tindall & Cox, London.
2. Department for Work and Pensions (2005) *Health, work and well-being – Caring for our future: A strategy for the health and well-being of working age people*, http://www.dwp. gov.uk/publications/dwp/2005/health_and_wellbeing.pdf last accessed 24.11.05.
3. Declaration of Human Rights, Article 23.
4. Chartered Institute of Personnel and Development (2005) *Occupational health and organisational effectiveness* www.cipd.co.uk last accessed 24.11.05.
5. Better Regulation Task Force (2004) Better Routes to Redress www.brtf.gov.uk last accessed 24.11.05.
6. Confederation of British Industry (2004) *Room for Improvement: absence and labour turnover 2004*. CBI, London.
7. World Health Organization (2002) *Good Practice in Occupational Health*.
8. Royal College of Nursing (2005); based on World Health Organization (2002) *Good Practice in Occupational Health*.
9. www.facoccmed. ac.uk

10. Nursing and Midwifery Council (2004) *Standards of Proficiency for Specialist Community Public Health Nurses*. NMC, London.
11. Royal College of Nursing (2005) *Competencies: An Integrated Career and Competency Framework for Occupational Health Nursing*. RCN, London.
12. British Occupational Hygiene Society www.bohs.org last accessed 24.11.05.
13. Ergonomics Society www.ergonomics.org.uk last accessed 24.11.05.
14. Institute of Occupational Safety and Health www.iosh.co.uk last accessed 24.11.05.
15. Chartered Institute of Physiotherapy www.csp.org.uk last accessed 24.11.05.
16. Nursing and Midwifery Council (2005) *Guidelines for Records and Record Keeping*. NMC, London.
17. General Medical Council (2001) *Standards of Practice*. GMC, London.
18. Tonnes, K. cited in Naidoo, J. & Wills, J. (2001) *Health Promotion: Foundations for Practice*, 2nd edn. Baillière Tindall, London.
19. Brennan, W. (2005) *Mental Wealth, Being Mentally Well* www.oliverbrennan.co.uk last accessed 24.11.05.
20. Brennan, W. (2005) Having a healthy mind. *Occupational Health* (Feb) **57** (2).
21. Mental Health Foundation (2003) Statistics on Mental Health Factsheet.
22. www.hse.gov.uk/stress/index.htm last accessed 02.12.05.
23. RR069 – *Evaluation of the Health and Safety (First-Aid) Regulations 1981 and the approved code of practice and guidance* www.hse.gov.uk last accessed 24.11.05.
24. Advisory, Conciliation and Arbitration Service (ACAS) Annual Report and Resource Accounts 2003/04.
25. Employment Act 2002.
26. Trades Union Congress (2000) *Focus on Health and Safety*. TUC, London.
27. Health and Safety Executive (1996) *Violence at Work* (IND(G)196L[rev 10/96]). HSE, London.

Chapter 5
In Sickness and in Health

Absence management

Absence management is the responsibility of company management, human resources and, of course, the individual staff member. Occupational health can play a very important part in advising and supporting management in helping to reduce absence rates and in promoting a healthy workforce. Indeed, the annual surveys into employee absence undertaken by the Chartered Institute of Personnel and Development (CIPD)[1] and the Confederation of British Industry (CBI)[2] confirm that the involvement of occupational health services is rated as the most effective method of managing long-term absence, despite its being only the fourth most commonly used approach to tackling the problem.

Firstly, it must be remembered that not all absence is unplanned or due to sickness, and that there are planned or scheduled absences, some of which are statutory rights and some of which are discretionary to the employment, such as:

- annual or study leave
- carers' leave
- maternity/paternity leave
- planned health care for surgery or other treatment
- public duties such as jury or military service
- trade union duties
- career breaks, sabbaticals, etc.

There have been various surveys and other research undertaken with regard to absence management, sickness absence and rehabilitation. There are many sources of statistics from studies and surveys, including the CIPD and CBI annual surveys, as noted above, and the Health and Safety Executive Occupational Health Statistics Bulletin.[3] The Occupational Health Statistics Bulletin deals mainly with work-related ill health, and the 2003/4 statistics show that over 2 million people in the UK suffer from ill health that they believe was caused, or made worse, by their current or past work. It goes on to say that over half the cases of work-related illness are based on musculoskeletal disorders, such as back pain or upper limb problems, or are related to stress and mental ill health.

The surveys generally indicate that the cost of absence to both the company and British industry is high. It is therefore sensible to assume that absence management is near to the top of many employers' lists of priorities. The focus of the absence management objectives are to reduce levels of absence by having in place sensible measures to prevent unplanned absence and improve attendance.

According to the 2004 Department of Health document *Choosing Health: making healthier choices easier*, 'being off work damages health and shortens life': a key issue for employers and employees is to try to prevent ill health, and to rehabilitate those who are sick back to participate in society and be a part of a workplace team.

Absence management policies and procedures are key to having an efficient system that staff can follow and understand. Developing these policies is a team effort and involves stakeholder representatives from:

- human resources/personnel
- senior and line managers
- employees and trade unions
- occupational health

Guidance for developing suitable policies and procedures is readily available and can be found in a number of publications:

Chartered Institute of Personnel and Development (2004) Absence Management Fact Sheet.
Walters, M. (2005) *The One-stop Guide to Absence Management*, Personnel Today Management Resources.
Health and Safety Executive (2004) *Managing Sickness Absence and Return to Work: An Employer's and Manager's Guide*, HSG 249, HSE.

A chart showing the flow of managing absence can be seen in Fig. 5.1.

Confidentiality

It is an essential part of the policy that the confidential nature of occupational health is considered and management's commitment to observing that confidentiality respected. Like all doctors and qualified nurses, occupational health professionals are covered by professional codes of conduct. This means that if patient confidentiality is breached, it is a professional conduct matter. As well as facing disciplinary action by their employer, they could be struck off the register and barred from practising within their profession. The occupational health professional's role is to advise employers of the fitness of an individual to work, his or her functional capacity and, where necessary, what adaptations need to be made to the work or the workstation to accommodate temporary or permanent disability, and also to offer a prognosis. There is often no need for employers to know the diagnosis and, should it be necessary to divulge this, the patient/client will need to give written permission for the information to be released. The professional governing bodies for nursing and medicine produce guidance on the ethical and professional conduct matters that relate to confidentiality.[4,5] (See also Chapter 2, concerning records and reports.)

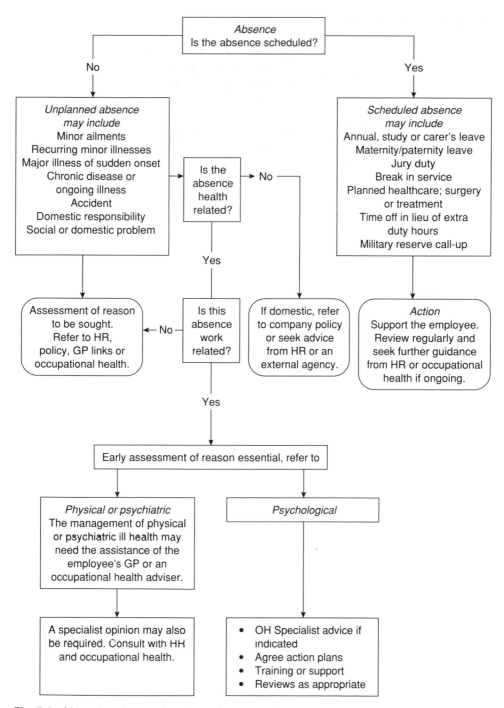

Fig. 5.1 Managing absence flow chart. Courtesy of www.manageabsence.com.

Handling sickness and absence

The cost of workplace sickness and absence is high. It is a major burden to employers; employees may lose pay depending on their contractual rights and the amount of time they are absent; state benefits and medical services cost taxpayers both directly and indirectly.

There is, as a result, a compelling drive on the part of employers and government to reduce the cost of absence, and to promote work rehabilitation as a cornerstone of achieving the aims. The Department for Work and Pensions (DWP) produced a UK Framework for Vocational Rehabilitation in October 2004, which says that statistics show that 'although there has been no worsening of health in the UK since the 1980s . . . sickness absence remains an issue'.[6] The DWP statistics indicate the following key points of note:

- An estimated 2–3% of the working population is off sick every day in the UK. Some 40 million working days a year are lost as a result.
- Many workers off because of sickness return after a matter of days. Others, on longer-term absence, account for a greater proportion of working time and cost.
- Around a quarter of GP consultations are work related.
- Around 7.6% of the working-age population claim incapacity benefits.
- Some 6.9 million people of working age self-report themselves as being long-term disabled. Around 5.4 million declare a work-limiting disability, with approximately half of those being in employment. About 46% of people with a declared disability are classed as economically active.

With employment rights in place to prevent discrimination on the grounds of disability and age, and the government's strategic plan to address demographic changes within the working population, employers must be ready to face a changing workforce profile and new employment policy challenges. The focus on occupational health is highlighted by these factors. There is a strong business case for effective and timely use of an occupational health service to address the goal of improving attendance levels. This is recognised by the NHS Plus initiative set up to provide an expert occupational health service to employers on a commercial basis. There is strong evidence that sickness and absence management is seen as effective when occupational health services are used, and yet still only some 62% of employers use the services.[1] Occupational health professionals can play a major part in helping to reduce sickness absence levels, managing work rehabilitation, and helping employers to comply with their legal obligations.

Handling sickness and absence requires particular management skills: these are sensitive issues, with many legal facets to consider in the process. Training those whose role encompasses this responsibility is vital. So too is an objective assessment as to whether individual managers have the time and skills to undertake the task. Not all managers do. There is also a convincing case for employers to appoint someone other than line management to handle the sensitive question of sickness and rehabilitation. Both the employee and the manager may feel that it is easier for this particular issue to be handled by a third party manager so that the working relationship is preserved when the other matters have been resolved.

Note that we have used the term 'third party manager' – this is not the occupational health professional. The role of occupational health is advisory in its specialist role as health professionals in the field of work. Occupational health, therefore, advises management in relation to health functionality and enabling matters, but should not be expected to make managerial decisions as these are not within the remit of its responsibility. Likewise, when a case is before an employment tribunal and occupational health provide evidence – for example, in a disability discrimination case – it will be for the tribunal to decide whether, on the basis of all the evidence they have heard, the employee is disabled within the meaning of the Act. In other words, it is for the occupational health professional to give the relevant health and medical reports, and then for the courts to decide on the legal conclusions to be drawn from the evidence.

Early referral to occupational health is essential and the importance of this cannot be stressed enough. Referral should be made on an appropriate form or letter and should be accompanied by a job description if the workplace cannot be visited by occupational health (see Appendix 4 for a management referral letter example and Appendices 5 to 9 for other useful and relevant sample letters and forms). There is certain information that is required by the occupational health service for every referral:

- Why is this person being referred?
- What has led up to this referral – sickness absence details, management concerns?
- Have they been informed?
- Have they given permission for the referral in some form – contract of employment/written authorisation?
- What is their job, and in what department do they work?
- What exactly does management want occupational health to advise upon?
- Any other relevant information.

From the occupational health perspective, it is important for health professionals to be given the relevant information about the workplace, duties, equipment, hours, etc. of the job. They will also need to be given details of any risk assessments that pertain to the job for which the person is employed. Sometimes occupational health may need to visit the workplace to ascertain the full facts, but employers should try to supply them with any relevant information in this respect when the initial referral is made.

One of the key issues in managing absence is to prevent the work-related sickness absence. There are two main causes of sickness absence that tend to predominate: musculoskeletal disorders and stress-related ill health. The occupational health team can help in the prevention of these conditions and support the rehabilitation of people back to work efficiently following sick leave.

Achieving improved attendance

In order to address the absence problem, employers need to keep good records, analyse and monitor these, and then have clear procedures for taking the appropriate action. Employers need to set standards and protocols on such matters as:

- sickness notification
- certification requirements
- keeping and measuring absence records
- return to work procedures
- medical reports
- taking account of the individual within a consistent and fair framework

While all sickness matters should be handled with the sympathy, understanding and compassion that tribunals expect of employers, the Employment Rights Act 1996 provides that termination of employment on the grounds of capability to do the job is a fair reason for dismissal. This can operate in a number of ways: the employee's illness may make it unsafe for him or her to continue in the employment; or frequent short-term absence can result in a disciplinary process focused on the conduct of the employee; or short-term absences with an underlying medical cause or long-term absence may entitle the employer to conclude that the employee is no longer capable of carrying out the work she or he was employed to do.

Absenteeism in the employment situation can refer to unauthorised absence or the more difficult to prove, and therefore to handle, cases that concern 'malingering', meaning falsely claiming to be ill. The latter would be treated as disciplinary matters by reason of misconduct but can be very difficult to prove, especially when the absence is supported by medical certificates. Absence records should differentiate between unauthorised absence and authorised absence for family leave, compassionate or other reasons that are not related to sick leave but are nonetheless legitimate and, in some cases, statutory.

Genuine sickness should not be treated as malingering. An employee cannot help being ill, and for that reason sickness is treated by the courts as a no-fault capability issue both in longer-term ill health situations and in frequent short-term absence where there is an underlying medical reason. However, the need for employers to run their business is acknowledged so that attendance standards can be set to enable the business to function properly and cost-effectively. The key issues expected of employers are:

- To identify whether there is an underlying medical reason for sickness absence.
- To ascertain the prognosis for the condition.
- To take account of any disability adjustment considerations.
- To set standard trigger points for action.
- To communicate appropriately with the employee.
- To treat people fairly and consistently.

- To set standards and help employees to achieve them.
- To adhere to employment rights legislation.

Frequent short-term absence

Frequent, or persistent, short-term absence is handled in a different way from longer-term ill health situations. The starting point in all cases is proper reporting and recording systems.

Employees must know how and when to report absence, what types of leave are available to them, what their statutory leave rights are, and what the attendance management protocols are within the organisation.

Managers must know what the protocols are, and must handle them consistently and properly. All managers should be trained in dealing with these sensitive and confidential issues and evaluated as to their ability to carry out this function as required. Given the complexities of such matters, it is possible that there will, as previously noted, be circumstances in which some managers are not able to take on this responsibility, or where the staff relationship is best preserved by its being undertaken by a different manager. This may especially be the case in, for example, small teams or close working relationships.

Most people suffer occasional bouts of minor illness such as colds and flu, stomach upsets, toothache, etc. Different people are affected in different ways by these illnesses: some people will need to take time off work and others will not. Some people will recover more quickly than others. These factors do need to be taken into account in the absence management protocol because there are genuine individual differences and susceptibilities to be considered.

General factors to be considered include:

- Welcoming people back to work and carrying out return to work interviews have proved to be effective in absence management. These interviews, if conducted correctly as a welcome rather than as a disciplinary measure, help to identify problems at an early stage and enable employees to feel valued and missed.
- Prompt investigation into what the nature of the absence is will be vital. If it is properly reported sickness then the following pointers may be considered. If it is not sickness, it will need to be handled differently as a potential misconduct matter or by giving the employee guidance as to what other leave options there are for certain situations.
- Seeing the employee on their return to work. This is essential after any period of absence. The employee may need to have adjustments to help them return, they may have an overwhelmingly high workload that could result in a recovery setback, or there may be an underlying and potentially recurrent health problem to address.
- If there is an occupational health service, a referral should be made as soon as the policy or the individual circumstances warrant this. Opinion should be sought as to the prognosis for improved attendance and/or any underlying health problems that may prevent this.

- Employees should be told of the standard of attendance expected. This should be reviewed so that improvements are noted as well as any failure to make improvements.
- Any disability discrimination issues must be taken into account.
- Adjustments to work and work equipment should be considered where appropriate. Temporary arrangements for reduced hours or for some home working arrangements may be helpful and appropriate.
- Employees should be warned appropriately if their sickness and absence is putting their employment at risk. If the absence is not medically certified, or there are no underlying medical factors to consider, this may be a matter of 'conduct' to be handled – albeit with appropriate sympathy, compassion and understanding – under the disciplinary policy.

Sickness during disciplinary and other internal proceedings

A recurring problem for management is that of an employee going off sick during a disciplinary, grievance or appraisal process. There may be a tendency to regard this as a cynical means by which employees are trying to avoid 'facing the music'. On the other hand, an employee who is suffering from health problems, but has been soldiering on at work, may just be tipped over the edge and become ill as a result of any such formal proceedings. These are usually stressful situations for employees, but the question that needs to be handled carefully is whether there is a stress-related illness, or other type of ill health, that genuinely warrants delaying proceedings and, if so, for how long. In some cases delay may only exacerbate stress and anxiety, but in other situations an employee may be genuinely too ill to account properly for themselves. Each case will need to be judged on its own facts and circumstances, which will need to be investigated. Useful guidance on how to handle these situations is available from the following websites: www.acas.org.uk and www.dti.gov.uk.

Key to investigating a sickness-related delay to internal proceedings can be a referral to occupational health. An employee who is not well enough to attend work for their full duties may, nonetheless, be fit enough to attend a meeting. Indeed, this may help to alleviate undue worry and stress by completing the internal proceedings and moving on. But there are dangers for employers who press on with proceedings without taking heed of proper procedures, employment rights, medical certificates and advice from occupational health. A genuinely ill employee could suffer damage to his health that might result in legal action against the employer, and there could be a serious risk of the employer's being in breach of contract and/or statutory employment rights. Remember that a breach of the statutory procedures in disciplinary, grievance and appeals can result in a finding of automatically unfair dismissal and a compensatory tribunal award being increased by up to 50% for the failure to follow required procedural steps.

Occupational health should be asked for advice as to whether and when an employee who is on sick leave might be able to deal with an internal meeting. It may also be sensible to seek advice from occupational health concerning any reasonable adjustments that could be offered to support the employee while he is not well: perhaps offering to meet somewhere other than at the place of work (though home visits may not be advisable in these situations), or offering the employee the chance to provide input to, say, an investigation, by written submissions or via a representative who is authorised to speak on his behalf. These are important options that may lead to a short delay but will not defer matters indefinitely. For many employees there is anecdotal evidence that a major cause of stress for them in these situations is their perceived humiliation at being seen to attend a disciplinary hearing, and so flexibility and acknowledgement of these factors can assist everyone involved.

The kinds of issues and options to be considered in these circumstances include:

- Considering and taking advice on any health-related absence that prevents internal proceedings taking place.
- Establishing the rules for medical evidence requirements of employees who report sick during internal proceedings: for example, submission of a doctor's certificate being required from day 1 of any such absence.
- Offering alternatives to those suffering from stress-related illness linked to disciplinary or other proceedings.
- Setting the rules of occupational sick pay entitlement in these situations.
- Making policy and contractual clauses known to employees.
- Ensuring compliance with employment rights legislation.

Longer-term ill health absence

Where the sick leave relates to medically certified ill health, this is not usually an issue of conduct or other disciplinary matter. Nonetheless, as we detail further in Chapter 6, it is worth a reminder here that, should the employment be at risk, the employee must be formally warned of this, albeit not in a disciplinary sense that implies misconduct, and proper statutory procedures must be followed at all meetings with management.

There are some key aspects of good practice that management should follow in these longer-term ill health cases, in addition to those that apply to short-term absence:

- Keep regular contact between the employer and employee. Establish a range of means to do so within company policy and practice guidance.
- Ensure that appropriate medical reports are obtained from occupational health, the GP and/or treating specialist. The GP or specialist reports may have been obtained in confidence to occupational health, and the latter's report will be based on the information these other reports contain and occupational health's knowledge of work-related health factors. This range of reports is what a tribunal will usually expect of a good employer.
- Ensure that the employee is informed of his rights to consent or withhold consent, have access to the report, and request amendments to the report

(see Chapter 2). But also alert the employee to the fact that the employer, while acknowledging these rights, reserves its position to make its decisions based on the information available to the company when drawing its conclusions relating to the employee's health and future employment.

- On the basis of the report and prognosis, and the employee's views, the employer must consider with the employee the return to work plan options, adjustments, support, re-training, re-deployment, and any other matters relevant and appropriate to the individual situation.
- When the employee returns to work, the employer and employee must comply with any recommendations made and accepted: review, support and monitor the situation.
- Where appropriate, defer action to press for a return to work. There will be instances where an employee is going to be off sick for a fairly long time but is likely to return at some foreseeable point. For compassionate and medical reasons, these situations could and should be managed appropriately, where possible: for example, a temporary replacement could be made to cover the absence, as in the case of maternity leave appointments.

Disability discrimination

The Disability Discrimination Act 1995 (as amended) (DDA) is at the forefront of many employment considerations with regard to the management of sickness absence, workplace rehabilitation and general return to work plans. This is a correct approach and concern.

It is worth noting some key points at the outset of this section:

- People who are disabled are not necessarily ill. Indeed, many people with a genuinely health-disabling condition want to work, do not take extraordinary sickness and absence leave, and are loyal and long-serving employees. In many instances good employment practice is actually focused on their being 'enabled' rather than disabled. UK employment legislation is increasingly founded upon these principles.
- Discrimination on the grounds of a disability can be the subject of legal action, whether or not the employment has ended. It is occasionally a misconception that disability discrimination can only occur if an employee is rejected for a position at the recruitment stage or if he is dismissed from employment.
- Decisions relating to whether or not a person is disabled within the meaning of the Act, or conclusions as to what adjustments constitute those considered reasonable in that particular employment situation, are not the prerogative of the occupational health adviser. Rather, it is for the occupational health professional to make recommendations and give medical or health-related advice or opinion that in turn will enable management to make its own decision.

The Disability Discrimination Act 1995 came into force on 2 December 1996. There have been significant amendments to the original Act, including those that came into force in subsequent years. At its inception there was no DDA case law precedent but there was an extensive body of case law relating to comparable cases in other types of discrimination. There was also the unfair dismissal case law generally, and specifically that concerning ill-health related dismissals.

Good practice can now be given a very much clearer direction through development of the legal framework and evaluation of the case law. The key factors that emerge from the employment rights developments need to be translated into the practical standards required of good employment practice standards today.

DDA definitions

The statutory definition of disability discrimination is when:

'A person directly discriminates against a disabled person, if, on the ground of the disabled person's disability, he treats the disabled person less favourably than he treats or would treat a person not having that particular disability whose relevant circumstances, including his abilities are the same as, or not materially different from, those of the disabled person.'

A person has a disability according to the DDA if:

'He has a physical or mental impairment which has a substantial and long term adverse effect on his ability to carry out normal day to day activities'

Recent changes to the DDA that took effect from December 2005 include:

- Removal of the requirement that a mental illness must be 'clinically well recognised' before it can amount to a mental impairment.
- Amendment to the definition of 'disability', so that a person with HIV, certain types of cancer or multiple sclerosis is deemed to be disabled from the point of diagnosis.
- A positive duty on public bodies to promote equality of opportunity for disabled people.

The definition of harassment under the Act is when:

'A person subjects a disabled person to harassment where, for a reason which relates to the disabled person's disability, he engages in unwanted conduct which has the purpose or effect of:
  i. violating the disabled person's dignity; or
  ii. creating an intimidating, hostile, degrading, humiliating or offensive environment for him.'

Reasonable adjustments

Identifying the need for any adjustments in the work or workplace is essential. This consideration has to be borne in mind throughout the process of enabling disabled people to work or when rehabilitating ill-health absentees back into the workplace. There is an increased emphasis on the need to make reasonable adjustments because the justification defence (for failure to make the adjustments) in general no longer applies. The extent of the duty applies to all stages of the employment process (see the Disability Discrimination Act 1995 (Amendment) Regulations 2003; the Disability Discrimination (Employment) Regulations 1996; and the Disability Discrimination (Meaning of Disability) Regulations 1996).

Good management practice must be to start reasonable adjustment considerations from the outset of the employment process, i.e. from the recruitment stage as covered in Chapter 1. The duty to make reasonable adjustments extends to:

- Any arrangements made by or on behalf of the employer; or
- Any physical feature of the employer's premises.

The duty arises where arrangements or physical premises/equipment places the 'disabled person concerned at a substantial disadvantage in comparison with persons who are not disabled' at any stage during the course of employment.

The employer has a duty to consider reasonable adjustments when it knows, or could reasonably be expected to know, that a particular applicant has a disability and is likely to be substantially disadvantaged. Monitoring sickness and absence trends within the organisation as a whole and by reference to the individual is therefore essential. An employer cannot claim that he knew nothing of a person's disability if there is, for example, an absence record that shows regular sickness patterns indicating that an underlying medical cause might exist. Failure to keep records or to examine them would not be a viable defence.

An 'unknown' health problem is often revealed as having been perfectly clear as identifiable to a reasonable employer when all the facts are examined. Absence records are often key to this. Tribunals look to evidence of a disability in four main areas:

- Does the person have an impairment?
- Does this have an adverse effect on that person's ability to carry out normal day-to-day activities?
- Is the adverse effect substantial?
- Is the adverse effect long term?

Impairment is taken to affect the ability to carry out normal day-to-day activities if it affects:

- mobility
- manual dexterity
- physical co-ordination
- continence
- ability to lift, carry or otherwise move everyday objects
- speech, hearing or eyesight
- memory or ability to concentrate, learn or understand
- perception of the risk of physical danger

Exclusions from the definition of impairment currently include:

- Addiction to or dependency on alcohol, nicotine, or any other substance (other than as a result of it being medically prescribed).

- Tendency to set fires; to steal; to physical or sexual abuse of other persons; exhibitionism; voyeurism.
- Seasonal allergic rhinitis (hay fever) except to the extent that it aggravates the effect of another condition.

Long-term impairment is defined as that which:

- Has lasted at least twelve months; or
- Is likely to last at least twelve months; or
- Is likely to last for the lifetime of the person; or
- Has ceased to have a substantial effect but is likely to recur.

The DDA provides examples of the kinds of adjustments an employer may be required to make:

- adjustments to premises
- allocating some of the disabled person's duties to another person
- transferring to another vacancy
- altering working hours
- assigning to a different workplace
- allowing absence for rehabilitation, assessment or treatment
- training
- acquiring or modifying equipment
- modifying instructions or reference manuals
- modifying procedures for testing or assessment
- providing a reader or interpreter
- providing supervision

Reasonableness

This is a word that is the subject of constant legal argument and interpretation. Under the DDA, what may be considered as reasonable in the circumstances will take into account:

- the effect of steps taken
- practicability
- cost and disruption
- employer resources

Case law

Risk assessment

The importance of risk assessment in all medical cases is clear. In *Jones* v. *Post Office* [2001] ICR 805, an insulin-dependent diabetic postman was removed from driving duties after the employer carried out a full and proper risk assessment. Although the tribunal did not agree with the employer's actions, the Court of Appeal did. They highlighted the importance of the properly conducted risk assessment in giving their decision.

Cont.

Knowledge of disability

This is a question that frequently arises. There is a wealth of case law that indicates the correct line to follow, albeit that each case will turn on its individual merits and facts.

The duty to make reasonable adjustments does not arise if the employer could not reasonably be expected to know that a person is disabled. But this does not mean that the employee needs to formally announce a disability.

In *O'Neill* v. *Symm and Company Ltd* [1998] ICR 481, the employee was dismissed because of sickness and absence after three months in the job. She had been diagnosed as suffering from ME (myalgic encephalopathy), but she did not tell her employers. The employers found Ms O'Neill to have been an efficient employee, and they had no indication that she suffered from any symptoms to lead them to believe they needed to make further enquiries. In upholding the employer's decision to dismiss her, the EAT took account of the Code of Practice, which states: 'The Act does not prevent a disabled person keeping a disability confidential from an employer. But this is likely to mean that unless the employer could reasonably be expected to know about the person's disability anyway, the employer would not be under a duty to make a reasonable adjustment. If a disabled person expects an employer to make a reasonable adjustment, then he will need to provide the employer – or, as the case may be, someone acting on the employer's behalf – with sufficient information to carry out that adjustment.'[7]

Reasonableness

Again, this is a matter that is regularly considered in individual cases and is a question of judicial interpretation depending on the facts and merits presented. The requirement upon employers is that they genuinely consider making reasonable adjustments and are able to evidence their efforts as having done so. In *Rossiter* v. *County Durham Magistrates' Courts* (1999) ET Case No. 2502425/99, Ms Rossiter's dismissal was held to have been fair when the employer sacked her for her poor attendance. She took frequent short-term absences, which were accepted as being for genuine health reasons albeit that there appeared to be no underlying medical cause for them. There were, however, a series of quite serious underlying personal problems that contributed to the problem significantly. But the tribunal held that the employer's business needs and the employee's needs could not be balanced so as to allow adjustments that would be reasonable in this case. The employer had done its best to assist Ms Rossiter and to support her for a significant time in an effort to allow her to recover, but the point of no return had been reached and no more could be expected of the employer.

Sickness absence management

In 2004 the CBI published its findings in a comprehensive absence and labour turnover survey undertaken with AXA.[2] The survey revealed that the most common cause of sickness absence was short-term illnesses such as colds and flu. The next most prevalent cause was recurring illness; in the case of manual workers this was exampled as back pain, and in non-manual workers as stress-related illness.

In these key areas of absence management, there are clear occupational health initiatives to be considered as potentially effective means by which absence for these reasons could be reduced, including for example:

- Sickness and absence management policy.
- Set protocols for recording and measuring absence. A useful guide as to how to do this is provided by ACAS: see www.acas.org.uk – Absence and Labour Turnover.
- Training appropriately skilled managers to handle the policy effectively.
- Return to work action protocols.
- Communications with employees on sick leave.
- Setting targets and measuring achievements – fairly and with due sensitivity.
- Rehabilitation planning: enabling adjustments and setting goals.
- Stress management risk assessments.
- Stress-reduction initiatives.
- Manual handling and ergonomics reviews.
- Training needs analysis.
- Physiotherapy service provision.
- Counselling service provision.
- Personal security information.
- Health promotion and information.

Employment policies and protocols

The importance of having clear policies cannot be overemphasised. They ensure fairness and consistency of treatment of all staff as well as providing a standard level for good and informed management practice. Evidence of fairness and consistency is an important factor in tribunal judgments.

Protocols through which managers can be guided as to how they should apply the employment policy are also essential. For example:

- Standard trigger points at which staff will be consulted.
- Manner of consultative meetings.
- Proper representation rights.
- Respecting privacy and permission
- Obtaining and safe keeping of medical evidence.
- Safeguarding employee health – related employment policies: drugs and alcohol, smoking, health.

There is a wealth of case law that shows employers examples of good practice and the proper standards expected of them in managing sickness absence. One of the key cases is that of *East Lindsey District Council* v. *Daubney* [1977] ICR 566, to which we shall return in Chapter 6. Although the case was heard before the DDA was in force, its principles remain important in absence management generally and specifically in relation to long-term ill health. Part of its general principles set a standard action plan for employers to follow:

- Consultation with employee.
- Medical investigation.
- Consideration of alternative employment. Today, having regard to the DDA, this consideration must include reasonable adjustments.

Another leading case that still sets the standard for fairness and reasonableness in managing ill health in employment is that of *Lynock* v. *Cereal Packaging Ltd* [1988] 1 CR, 670 EAT:

- Genuine illness is not to be treated as a disciplinary matter.
- Handle each case with sympathy, understanding and compassion.
- The 'warning' system in disciplinary situations to be dealt with as 'caution' when the stage is nearing where, with the best will in the world, continued employment is at risk.

This case provided important guidance for getting people back to work safely so that any fears that the employee has about his return should either be resolved or be capable of resolution one way or another. Practical steps to achieve this include:

- Review of the absence records.
- Compare these with others within the department, and with the absence records of other departments.
- Check steps taken by management or human resources: telephone calls, letters, personal visits.
- Consider medical reports. These should be current and include an occupational health report and any treating specialist's reports. A GP report may also be appropriate. Relevant and timely reports are important to both long-term sickness and frequent short-term absence situations.
- Review whether there is a need for a further medical report or opinion on adjustments for the employee's return to work.
- Invite the employee to a meeting at work or consider a meeting off site, depending upon the individual circumstances. Home visits are not always appropriate from the perspective of the manager or the employee. An off-site meeting – perhaps over coffee or lunch – is often well received. But coming back to the workplace for a meeting can also be helpful sometimes in 'breaking the ice' for the return to work.
- Return to work assessment may need to cover stress factors including domestic stressors.
- Physical factors should be taken into account: for example, is an ergonomic assessment needed?
- Employee participation should be sought in the risk assessment and evaluation process of rehabilitation and absence management.

Return to work policy

The employer should have a policy on dealing with the return to work of short-term and long-term absentees. In addition to applying it evenly and with a view to making reasonable adjustments to comply with the DDA, the employer should update the policy regularly, particularly if needs are shown to arise in risk assessments. The policy should reflect the paramount needs of the business to run efficiently and the need for staff cooperation.

The recovery of a seriously ill or injured person may be slow but helped by the knowledge that there is a supportive employer who is sensitive to the individual circumstances as well as to the needs of the business. Rehabilitation is not just a simple employment issue but part of a complex team effort involving occupational health professionals, general managers and human resources. There will be close liaison between these people and the individual employee. This should continue throughout the preparation for return to work, which could be on a phased basis, and through the establishment of a temporary or permanent change of working pattern.

Return to work: the occupational health perspective

Excellent guidance on rehabilitation is given by Waddell and Burton in their *Concepts of Rehabilitation for the Management of Common Health Problems*.[8] Much of their work is based on the bio-psychosocial model of disability where rehabilitation needs to address all the biological, personal and psychological, and social dimensions. This is similar to the adaptation model for nursing introduced by Sister Callista Roy in the 1960s.[9] The *International Classification of Functioning Disability and Health*[10] is also based on the bio-psychosocial model following research, and so it is widely accepted.

Occupational health may well recommend a phased return to work. To start the process after a long period of absence, they may also suggest that the first step could be to invite the employee for an informal meeting with colleagues by way of reintroduction to the workplace, in order to break the ice and enable the employee to note any significant changes. In *Tolleys Guide to Employee Rehabilitation*[11] it is suggested that a return to work programme might include:

- A minimum of 16 hours per week worked.
- A minimum of 4 hours per day worked.
- A gradual increase of hours over 6–8 weeks.
- Regular review by occupational health.
- All rehabilitation therapeutics, such as physiotherapy or counselling, to be taken outside working hours where possible.

Returning to the legal perspectives, it is important for the employee to have access to any additional training and support for as long as he needs it, subject to the requirements of the business to be able to function. In other words, the rehabilitation process should be managed within the parameters of reasonable adjustments.

The rehabilitation process places a heavy burden on the OH practitioner to assess what is, what might have been and what should be in place to encourage the absentee back to work. Although the needs of the business must be satisfied, the employer must be able to assure the returning employee that his recovery will not be impeded, nor will he be at risk of a work-related relapse, or even a worsening of his condition. Whatever steps are taken to enable the rehabilitation process and the return to work, the workplace must be safe and the employee fit to return. Health and safety is the overriding factor in these considerations. Whether the employee is disabled or suffering from an isolated bout of ill health, the risk of relapse must be considered.

Case law

Returning to the judgment in *Lynock* v. *Cereal Packaging Ltd* [1988] 1 CR 670 EAT, the judge stated the way in which employers can properly approach their management of sickness absence:

> 'The approach of an employer in this situation is, in our view, one to be based on . . . three words . . . sympathy, understanding and compassion . . . one has to look at the whole history and the whole picture . . . every case must depend upon its own facts, and provided that the approach is right, the factors which may prove important to an employer in reaching what must inevitably have been a difficult decision, include perhaps some of the following – the nature of the illness; the likelihood of it recurring or some other illness arising; the length of the various absences and the spaces of good health between them; the need of the employer for the work done by the particular employee; the impact of the absences on others who work with the employee; the adoption and the exercise of carrying out the policy; the important emphasis on a personal assessment of the ultimate decision and, of course, the extent to which the difficulty of the situation and the position of the employer has been made clear to the employee so that the employee realises that the point of no return, the moment when the decision was ultimately being made may be approaching. These, we emphasise are not cases for disciplinary approaches; these are for approaches of understanding.'

In addition to the above, employers must now also take account of disability discrimination issues and the following of statutory procedures but otherwise the case remains a cornerstone for establishing management protocols for best practice handling of sickness absence.

In *Freer Bouskell* v. *Brewer* (2004) UKEAT/377/03, Ms Brewer was a legal secretary who suffered from claustrophobia. Her desk was moved from a spacious office to a cramped one because the employer needed the old room for conferences. She had a serious panic attack and fled the building. The employers ignored her GP's letter explaining the nature of her illness and requesting adjustments by way of seating her in a more spacious area. Ms Brewer resigned and claimed constructive dismissal and disability discrimination. She succeeded. The dismissal was upheld as fair. Freer Bouskell had contributed to the employee's illness by making her move to a cramped office when it knew about her condition and that it could be exacerbated. Further, Ms Brewer's conduct was not blameworthy in that she had not sought psychiatric help for her long-standing condition. It is worth noting that since this case was heard the statutory dispute procedures have come into force requiring, since 1 October 2004, employees and employers to utilise proper internal proceedings in an effort to raise and settle a grievance of this nature.

Sick pay and medical evidence

The question of medical evidence of illness is not always straightforward. This is partly due to there being two sets of rules as to what constitutes proper medical evidence required by an employer: the statutory sick pay (SSP) rules, and the contractual requirements of the employer for any company sick pay provisions they offer. The rules need not be the same, but the statutory rules cannot be varied for SSP payment qualification purposes.

As part of the terms and conditions of service, employers usually have their own rules about notification and certification, and in particular for qualifying for occupational sick pay (OSP) – the company sick pay scheme. These could include the method, timing and frequency of contact required, the person to notify, when and where to send medical certificates, any rules concerning self-certification and medical certification, and what can happen if employees do not adhere to the internal rules. Failure to follow company rules cannot result in any alteration to SSP entitlement, however, unless the SSP rules themselves have been breached.

Statutory sick pay

Dealing first with the SSP regulations, some certification is normally required from the fourth day of absence onwards. Self-certification is required for periods of up to one week and medical certificates for longer than this. What constitutes a 'medical certificate' for SSP purposes covers a broader scope than some employers are prepared to accept for their OSP rules. That is perfectly lawful for OSP purposes, but employers must comply with acceptance of one of the approved types of medical certificate for SSP purposes.

Advice and guidance on SSP generally, including medical certification, is available from various official sources: see www.acas.org.uk (Absence and Labour Turnover) and the Department for Work and Pensions (formerly the Department of Social Security) www.dwp.gov.uk. These tend to be rather general as to what constitutes a medical certificate, stating for example that a doctor's note is usually what employers require. The most definitive guidance[12] comes from HM Revenue and Customs (formerly Inland Revenue), which administers the SSP payments system and states the rules for payment and qualification, including medical certification: see www.hmrc.gov.uk. In the Conditions of Entitlement section for employers it is noted that an employer *cannot* for SSP purposes require employees to notify:

- the employer in person
- earlier than the first day of sickness
- by a specific time
- more often than once a week
- on a special form
- on a medical certificate

The rules go on to state in the terms and conditions covering Evidence of Incapacity for Work (section 5) that employers are entitled to ask employees to provide 'reasonable evidence of incapacity such as a doctor's statement' after the first seven days of a spell of sickness. Self-certification is used for spells of between four and seven days. The terms and conditions of SSP also state:

- That a doctor's statement is strong evidence of incapacity and should usually be accepted as conclusive unless there is very strong evidence to the contrary.

Although this rule applies to SSP, it is a matter that is, we suggest, general best practice. It is sometimes true that a GP may be less well able to advise on work-related health issues than an occupational health specialist, but this is usually an issue best resolved by doctor to doctor discussions in order to try to agree a way forward.

Returning to SSP, the rules of medical certification bring a further complication as to what, for SSP purposes, constitutes a certificate. Here, the rules are that such certificate need not be from a registered medical practitioner. Employers are told that they must consider these non-medical practitioner certificates 'on their merits'. Examples are given of other types of certificates from people such as osteopaths, chiropractors, Christian scientists, herbalists and acupuncturists, but it is for the employer to decide whether these are acceptable certifications even for SSP. Good practice suggests that employees be told in their terms and conditions of employment and/or the sickness and absence policy what the employer finds acceptable as medical certification: for example, 'A medical certificate is generally expected from the employee's doctor but could where appropriate be accepted from a chartered physiotherapist who is treating the employee, for a stated limited period, after which time a certificate from a medical practitioner is required.'

The key point is that the employee should know in advance what is acceptable. This applies to the sickness reporting rules in general too: there is nothing to prevent an employer asking that sickness be reported by a certain time to a named manager, for example. This makes it clear to the responsible employee what is expected of him, and it greatly assists the employer's management of the work. The important point for SSP compliance is that where an employee does not, for example, report sick by the required time, their SSP payment should not be stopped even if their OSP is not allowed because of the failure to adhere to company rules.

Occupational sick pay

Employers can have their own rules about certification for all sickness absence or for the entitlement to OSP. The SSP guidance will be relevant though not obligatory in this respect. It is generally good practice to have the same basic rules for both types of payment but it is also possible for an employee to qualify for SSP but not OSP where the rules are more stringently set by the employer.

Some employers require medical certificates for all sickness absence for the company sick pay rules, even though this is likely to be costly for employees because doctors usually charge for this service. Some employers require a doctor's certificate for any absence once a certain level of absenteeism has been reached – for example, after more than two periods of sickness in a six-month period. Some employers require medical certificates covering any sickness absence, of whatever duration, preceding or following bank holidays or holiday, or for any absence for illness that delays disciplinary or other internal proceedings. There are often specific rules covering sickness that occurs during holiday and vice versa that will need to be made clear in the terms and conditions of employment. The question as to how foreign medical certificates are regarded by the employer should also be made clear in employment information and policy. Further information and guidance is available from ACAS publications.[13]

There are many types of OSP schemes involving differing levels and length of payments. SSP lasts for up to 28 weeks but OSP will have differing terms and conditions. It is of course not obligatory on employers to offer OSP at all, but most larger employers do so. The details of the occupational sick pay scheme should be notified to employees in their written statement of terms of employment (their contract), which should set out entitlements to company sick pay and the rules with which employees have to comply in order to qualify for payments. Details should include levels of payment, for how long payments will last, any qualifying conditions such as length of service, any re-qualifying conditions once entitlement is exhausted, and the relationship between sickness and holidays.

Likewise, as was mentioned earlier in this section, some employers make it a term and condition of employment that OSP be limited or suspended during disciplinary proceedings. If this is the case then those terms and conditions need to be carefully drafted and made known to staff through the relevant policy documents and their contract of employment. If an employee is suspended pending a disciplinary matter that involves a serious misconduct allegation, the suspension will be on full pay but subject to certain terms and conditions. These will cover being available during normal working times, and should also make provision for any need to take sick leave and holiday that may occur during this time, how it will be treated and notified, etc. The terms and conditions of employment should also refer to company policy on other health-related issues such as alcohol and drugs policies and medical suspensions.

When employees return to work on a temporarily part-time basis as part of a rehabilitation process, the terms and conditions of service to cover what happens to pay in these circumstances should be clear and consistent. For example, some employers pay only the hours worked, some pay at full salary for a limited time, and some make up part or all of the difference in pay through OSP entitlement. If a permanent change in hours, duty or location takes place following a return to work after illness, an agreed contractual change will be necessary.

It is sensible for employers to state company policy on occupational health referrals and medical examinations. A general clause covering this should be contractual and might be worded along the following lines:

'The Company reserves the right to require employees to be referred to an occupational health service and/or to undergo a medical examination by a doctor, appointed by the Company, at any stage during his/her employment and during any period of absence. In the event of a serious, prolonged or recurrent illness, or if the Company has cause for concern regarding the employee's fitness to carry out his/her duties, the Company may request the employee to attend an occupational health service and/or an independent doctor for a medical examination to assess his/her medical condition or fitness for work. The employee will be required to give his/her consent to a report being sent to the Company concerning his/her fitness or otherwise to work or on any other relevant health related matter.'

Medical suspension

A medical suspension must be for a genuine reason certified by a medical practitioner who is not necessarily the employee's GP. Depending upon the nature of the business and the duties of the employee, such suspensions may sometimes be necessary or even mandatory. See the Public Health (Control of Disease) Act 1984 and the Public Health (Infectious Diseases) Regulations 1998 SI No. 1546. Some jobs, for example those involving exposure to ionising radiation, lead and certain other hazardous substances, are covered under special health and safety regulations. Pregnant women are also protected by legislation, including medical suspension rules, where their own health or that of the unborn child could be put at risk as a result of working conditions. Specific guidance on these situations is available from the DTI or HSE web sites on www.dti.gov.uk or www.hse.gov.uk.

In certain circumstances, as exampled, an employee who might ordinarily be able to work may be suspended under the mandatory regulations. The Employment Rights Act 1996 provides that most employees who are suspended under these regulations have the right to be paid for a limited period of the suspension.

There can be other circumstances when an employer considers that medical suspension is necessary, usually on the advice of occupational health or a doctor: for example, in food handling jobs or in certain health professions. In these situations it can sometimes be appropriate to ask the employee, who is otherwise fit and well enough, to undertake different duties for a time. Employment policy protocols should cover these situations, and the terms and conditions of employment should also include provision for them.

It is worth noting the fact that where an employee is found to have tested HIV positive or is known to be suffering from AIDS, this is not a reason for suspending that person from work, or for changing their duties arbitrarily, or for terminating their employment. Guidance as to these situations and the actions appropriate to specific situations can be found on various respected authority websites, including the HSE and ACAS as previously quoted, and the Terrence Higgins Trust on www.tht.org.uk.

Musculoskeletal disorders

Occupational health perspective

Musculoskeletal disorders cover a wide range of ill health and injuries, the most prevalent of which are back injuries and upper limb disorders. The Health and Safety Executive say that musculoskeletal disorders (MSDs) are the most common occupational illness in the UK, affecting some 1 million people a year. They include problems such as low back pain, joint injuries and repetitive strain injuries of various sorts. It is thought that some 60 to 80% of people suffer with back pain at some time, but many carry on, take a few analgesics and recover in a few days or weeks, while others go on to develop long-term problems.

Back injury and work-related upper limb disorders (WRULDs), a sub-section of MSDs, are broad classifications and refer to a series of health problems that are among the common, and often preventable, causes of sickness absence. The Health and Safety Commission strategy for tackling WRULDs is clearly explored in their book *Upper Limb Disorders in the Workplace* (HSG 60 rev.), which aims to help with the prevention and reduction of MSDs and working days lost in accordance with the targets set in *Securing Health Together*.[14]

Despite every effort, there will always be those who do suffer with back problems. A very useful resource for health professionals to recommend or give to patients/clients is *The Back Book: the Best Way to Deal with Back Pain*,[15] which contains the latest thinking on back pain and is based on proper research. It is written by a team of leading UK experts who encourage people to get active and return to normal living.

Painful musculoskeletal conditions, long-term absence and disability can be prevented by employers undertaking suitable risk assessments of employee workstations and manual handling, and putting in place appropriate control measures as required by various pieces of legislation and Health and Safety Executive guidance.

- *Management of Health and Safety at Work Regulations 1999 Approved Code of Practice and Guidance* L21 (HSE 1999a)
- *Work with Display Screen Equipment: Guidance on the Regulations* (HSE 2003)
- *Safe Use of Work Equipment: Approved Code of Practice and Guidance* L22 (HSE 1998)
- *Manual Handling: Guidance on Regulations* L23 (HSE 2004).

The regulations establish a hierarchy of measures:

(a) To avoid hazardous manual handling operations as far as is reasonably practicable. The guidance suggest such controls as redesigning the task, automation or mechanising the process, and these follow the control measures also outlined in MHSWR, under regulation 4.
(b) To undertake suitable and sufficient assessment of any hazardous manual handling that cannot be avoided.
(c) To reduce the risk, again following (a) above.

In order to do this the acronym **TOIL** is useful, where:

- **T is for task**: What is the actual work? Is it at a work station? What has to be lifted or moved to where? Are there any obstacles in the way? Is it a difficult or dangerous route to move?
- **O is for organisation** or environment: Where is this happening – inside or out? Factory or office? Who else is there? Public or other workers, etc.?
- **I is for individual**: Are they suitable and fit for the task? Do they understand what they should be doing? Have they received appropriate information and training?
- **L is for load**: Consider not just the weight but more importantly the size and shape as well as the consistency, smooth or rough, hot or cold, etc.

Employment law perspectives

In the 1990s there was what seemed at times to be almost an epidemic of WRULD or RSI (repetitive strain injury) related damages claims being reported in the news. A number of factors common to work-related injuries and diseases have combined to ensure that there is today a greater awareness of the problems and preventative measures that can help to reduce injury and associated litigation. This increased awareness does not diminish the importance or risk of the illness or injury, but a study of the legal processes in relation to WRULDs can provide some useful guidance as to handling the whole sphere of MSDs.

There is a risk of a WRULD when the nature of the work involves the use of:

- pounding or vibrating equipment such as drills
- hole-punching
- polishing gadgets
- household/builders' tools
- dental equipment
- repetitive movements such as in keyboard work or on a production line work.

Legal protection for proper and safe working practices is provided in criminal law under the Health and Safety at Work etc. Act 1974 and its subordinate legislation, in particular the Management of Health and Safety at Work Regulations 1999, which require risk assessments to be made. The employer is under a duty to provide a safe place and system of work and safe equipment, and employees also have a duty to take care of themselves. The need for risk assessment and health surveillance is paramount to meeting the obligations.

Under civil law, when an employee is injured or suffers an illness attributable to work equipment or working practice, there is a potential claim in negligence against the employer. The pivotal question will be that of whether the employer knew or ought to have known of the risk inherent in the work system. There may also be a related breach of contract claim for any alleged failure of the employer to keep a safe place and system of work.

Personal injury claims in English law include an element of general damages to compensate for pain, suffering and loss of amenity. There are other elements of damages that can be awarded to take account of the ongoing care and amenities of the person, which are assessed on an individual basis. The sums involved in the general damages amounts follow the Judicial Studies Board Guidelines in Personal Injury Cases, which include the following examples[16] in relation to MSDs and WRULDs:

Shoulder injuries
Severe: up to £26,000
Serious: up to £10,500
Moderate (e.g. frozen shoulder with limitation of movement): £4,250 to £7,000

Elbow injuries
Severely disabling: up to £26,500.
Moderate injuries include tennis elbow: usually in the region of £7000.

Wrist injuries
Complete loss of function: up to £33,000
Significant disability with limited movement: up to £21,500
Persistent pain and stiffness: up to £13,500
Recovery complete but over a protracted period: up to £5500

Hand–arm vibration syndrome (HAVS)/vibration white finger
Most serious: up to £21,000
Minor: up to £4750

Back injuries
Severely disabling: up to £93,000
Seriously disabling, such as including some impaired bladder and bowel function, severe sexual difficulties: in the region of £45,000
Continuing severe pain, other suffering or functional impairment: up to £38,000
Moderate: up to £21,500
Minor: up to £7500

Work-related upper limb disorders cover such conditions as:

Tenosynovitis: inflammation of synovial sheaths of tendons, resolving with rest over a short period. May lead to loss of grip and dexterity.

De Quervain's tenosynovitis: usually restricted to the thumb.

Stenosing tenosynovitis: 'trigger finger/thumb', thickening tendons.

Carpal tunnel syndrome: constriction of median nerve of the wrist or thickening of surrounding tissue. Surgery usually successful.

Epicondylitis: inflammation of the elbow joint (medial – golfer's elbow; lateral – tennis elbow).

The Health and Safety Executive issued new guidance to comply with revised legislation introduced by the Control of Vibration at Work Regulations 2005, which deal with the effects of vibration on the limbs and the whole body.[17] The guidance covers health surveillance and a revised guide for employers and occupational health professionals. There is a transitional period for the exposure limit values up to 2010. This would allow work activities where the use of older tools and machinery cannot keep exposures below the exposure limit value to continue in certain circumstances. The transitional period has been extended to 2014 in the case of whole-body exposures in the agriculture and forestry sectors.

The vibration may be subtle, as in the form of dental drills, or more obvious, such as the effects suffered by coal miners and road maintenance workers. Hand–arm vibration syndrome (HAVS) is one of the multitudes of disorders that affect people involved in the use of machinery or equipment that either requires repetitive movements on the part of the operator or subjects the limbs of the operator to transmitted movement.

The civil law has long imposed a duty of care on employers to ensure the health, safety and welfare of their employees in the workplace, and a correlative duty on the employees not to undertake tasks or go about their jobs in such a way as to risk their own health and safety or that of others. The common law duty, supported by the criminal law in the form of the Health and Safety at Work etc. Act 1974 and European derived Regulations, ensures that any employer who fails to provide a safe system of work and safe equipment will be liable to his employees who suffer injury as a result of that failure. The risk of injury must be reasonably foreseeable and, these days, should have been identified in a suitable and sufficient risk assessment under the Management of Health and Safety at Work Regulations. A risk that is not identifiable after a proper risk assessment may not have been reasonably foreseeable. The crucial factor is whether the employer knew or ought to have known of the risk and, if so, took reasonably practicable preventive steps.

The condition of writer's cramp has been known since man first took up the quill. Then came a work system involving rapid input of data into computers and a more intensive use of keyboards than was ever known in the typewriter age. The condition became known as RSI and was characterised by its seeming lack of connection with any formal, orthopaedic diagnosis, and in some cases a poor prognosis. The occupational health profession was and remains concerned about dealing with diffuse symptoms arising from similar work processes involving upper limb and hand activity in particular.

Before the main impact of risk assessments, there were indications that some employers appeared to be unable to recognise that human joints and muscles needed as much care and maintenance as the machinery or equipment that was causing injuries. But of great concern was the financial impact of the increasing volume of litigation. The civil damages claims that succeeded were those where a medical condition was identified and work-related causation proven to exist on the balance of probabilities.

The foundation of the prevention and mitigation of the occurrence of RSI, WRULD and back disorders is risk assessment. Employers who consider risk assessment based upon the business case and financial balance will take into account that:

- A conviction in the criminal court is likely to increase the injured person's chance of success in their civil claim.
- Any insurance cover will not cover fines imposed by the courts.
- Claims or prosecutions will affect insurance premiums.

Case law has helped provide employers with a set of guidelines to ameliorate the risk of RSI. A priority is the monitoring of workplace practices to test effectiveness, and to adapt or improve as indicated by the findings.

Case law

A clear guide to the prevention of RSI was provided by a well-known early claim that involved a group of chicken pluckers who contracted tenosynovitis as a result of their work. In *Mountenay (Hazzard) and Others* v. *Bernard Matthews* (1993), the judge set out the following guidelines for employers to follow to reduce the risk as far as reasonably practicable:

- Warn of the risk.
- Enable employees to make informed choice as to whether they will take the risk.
- Advise employees to take medical advice at the first sign of aching wrists or hands.
- Provide mechanical assistance for squeezing movements.
- Introduce new employees gradually to repetitive working movements.
- Rotate duties.

Employer checklist: a general guide to RSI monitoring

- Assess risk, reduce, prevent/ameliorate.
- New or improved equipment – proper usage, buying research, training.
- Is cessation of practice or new equipment feasible?
- Maintenance records checked.
- Training in ergonomics, posture, handling of tools, their proper usage – including the right tools for the right job.
- Compliance with health and safety legislation checked, including for example: Provision and Use of Work Equipment Regulations 1998 (PUWER 98), which came into force on 5 December 1998; Personal Protective Equipment at Work Regulations 1992 (PPE).
- Productivity.
- Health risk assessment.
- Health surveillance.

Employer checklist: work environment

- Proper ventilation and temperature for the work.
- PPE – clothing, gloves chairs, tables, arm rests.
- Proper training.
- Regular work breaks.
- Workstation ergonomics.
- Routine and as required health surveillance.
- Regular health checks – e.g. eye tests offered as appropriate.
- Health and safety inspections.
- Rotation of duties.
- Absence trends analysis.

Stress-related illness

It is current thinking that everyone's general health is affected by stress and could be improved by a reduction of stress levels. The HSE commissioned a study on the role of work stress and psychological factors in the development of musculoskeletal disorders in 2004.[18] The objectives of the study were to investigate factors that increased the likelihood of employees reporting high levels of perceived job stress, and whether job stress itself increased the likelihood of their reporting musculo-skeletal complaints. The report is useful background information to consider with other HSE publications that deal with the preventive aspects of stress disorders.

The HSE also provides guidance for employees and employers that aims to help both to take responsibility and action to tackle stress management. The guide, aimed at employees, offers insight into the causes of stress, why it should be dealt with and what to do about it.[19] Occupational health resources can greatly assist in dealing with concerns and can contribute to relevant risk assessments and design of stress reduction strategies.

Essentially, issues of concern should be jointly resolved between staff and management at the earliest opportunity. Staff need to be conversant with their responsibilities and the employment supports available to them so that they are aware of the need to comply with arrangements such as counselling or stress management training. Stress is unlikely to be a one-way process: employees should also be encouraged to help themselves wherever possible. Occupational health involvement can assist in helping to identify when stress may be imported from home. External causes of stress can affect perceptions of work-related problems and can also aggravate physical conditions.

The HSE, together with a number of organisations that include local authorities, ACAS, the CIPD and others, is working on a campaign to raise awareness of stress at work, and from this the HSE has produced the management standards.[19] These standards are based on research that showed that there are six key areas of work design that, if not properly managed, may lead to ill health, reduced productivity and increased sickness absence.[20] The HSE has identified six key areas and describes the standards that employers should try to attain.[21] In each area a risk assessment should be carried out to cover these points:

- *Demands:* the demands of the job – ensure that employees can cope.
- *Control:* the degree of employee control over their work – consult with employees so that they can have a say in how they should go about their work.
- *Support:* the level of management and colleague support provided – provide information and support through accessible policies and procedures – give regular and constructive feedback.
- *Relationships:* the quality of work relationships – this is a cue to become aware of and eliminate workplace intimidation and bullying.
- *Role:* employee role within the organisation and how it is managed – roles and responsibilities should be clearly defined.
- *Change:* the management of change – communication and involvement are key issues here.

In Appendix 10 we have provided a general template to use as a starting point for stress risk assessments based upon these six areas. This will need to be adapted for the organisation and department to take account of particular circumstances and availability of support services such as occupational health, human resources, counselling, etc.

An individual under stress is prone to illness of a physical or a psychological nature. Stress at work can relate to adverse psychosocial factors including difficulties with maintaining the confines of the job description, working too long hours, and having to cope with physical violence risk, verbal abuse or confrontation with members of the public. These matters can cause or exacerbate illness. Although management has no control over domestic matters, the workplace and system of work can be arranged so that problems can be resolved through general discussion and open procedures. Use of the statutory dispute resolution procedures, such as raising a grievance, could well be another element to consider in managing stress at work.

Case law: work-related stress

Work-related stress has also become the subject of litigation over recent years. In 2002 clarity was provided by case law in a series of enjoined case judgments.

The decision of the Court of Appeal in the joined cases of *Sutherland (Chairman of the Governors of St Thomas Becket RC High School)* v. *Hatton, Somerset County Council* v. *Barber*[22] and *Sandwell Metropolitan Council* v. *Jones and Baker Refractories Ltd* v. *Bishop* [2002] EWCA Civ 76 sets out some very important pointers for employers in the key preventive aspects of stress management, as well as in how to handle stress-related claims.

The judgment highlights key issues and important considerations for occupational health personnel and employers. It sets out clearly how employers should manage health and safety issues in general. Risk assessments should be based on standards that clarify a focus on the important principles as follows:

- There are no special control mechanisms for 'stress' – ordinary employer liability applies.
- The employer will be liable if the harm was reasonably foreseeable.
- Subject to causation, there must be an identifiable injury to health (i.e. a diagnosed illness).
- Causation must be established: any diagnosed illness must be attributable to stress at work.
- The court will look at what the employer knew or ought to have known about the alleged stress factors.
- Foreseeability depends on what the employer knows or ought to have known about the individual. It may be harder to foresee mental disorders than physical, unless other factors pertain, such as known vulnerability.
- The test applies whatever the occupation.
- Risk assessments should cover objective and subjective criteria (that is, covering the perspective of both employer and employee).

Six cases concerning employers' liability for work-induced stress-related illness were joined for their hearing at the Court of Appeal and are of particular importance in guiding best practice: *Hartman* v. *South Essex Mental Health and Community Care NHS Trust; Best* v. *Staffordshire University; Wheeldon* v. *HSBC Bank Ltd; Green* v. *Grimsby & Scunthorpe Newspapers Ltd; Moore* v. *Welwyn Components Ltd; Melville* v. *Home Office* [2005] IRLR 293.

Cont.

Their route started in the High Court, which decided in favour of five of the employee/claimants. All the losers appealed, with the result that the Court of Appeal overturned three of the decisions that had been in favour of the employees.

The question for the Court of Appeal to decide was that of employers' liability for psychiatric injury alleged to have been caused to employees by work-related stress. A central issue was whether the employer should have reasonably foreseen that staff would be prone to the illnesses, to which they in fact succumbed, if they followed the work arrangements imposed on them.

Cases coming to court now will also have consideration given to the use of practical elements of the HSE guidelines. The legal test applied by the courts is one that can easily be put into practice to forestall or defend personal injury claims, whether for psychological or physical harm: 'is the standard of care taken by the employer that which would be offered by a reasonable and prudent employer taking positive thought for his workers' safety in light of what he ought to know?'.

The two successful employees in the Court of Appeal

Applying the test of the reasonably prudent employer, the Court of Appeal found that in *Wheeldon* v. *HSBC Bank Ltd* the facts indicated that the employer was liable for the employee's depressive illness. HSBC's occupational health team had reported that Wheeldon's depression had been precipitated by work factors and advised that steps should be taken to deal with these issues. A reasonably prudent employer would have taken such steps. HSBC's failure to do so meant that they were liable for having caused the illness.

In *Melville* v. *Home Office*, Melville succeeded in the High Court, whose decision was upheld by the Court of Appeal, again on the specific facts. Melville was a prison officer whose duties included dealing with the bodies of prisoners who had committed suicide. The prison service had policies to deal with the approach to psychological trauma arising from these sorts of incidents, which happen from time to time in the prison service; in other words, these events were reasonably foreseeable, as was the harm that was likely to ensue. Not only did it have the policies and procedures, but there was counselling available to deal with the aftermath of these incidents. However, the failure to implement its systems meant that, when the officer became ill, the employer was held to be liable. In the decision, it was noted that the availability of an occupational health counselling service is not necessarily conclusive evidence that the employer has foreseen that psychiatric injury will occur, but having occupational health services available means that the employer is in a position to be able to comply with the duty of care to ensure the well-being of the employee.

The losing parties

In the *Hartman* v. *South Essex Mental Health and Community Care NHS Trust* case, the employee disclosed previous mental health problems to the occupational health department of the employing NHS Trust. As the information was confidential, the employer could not be deemed to have knowledge of risk of further psychiatric injury. The Court of Appeal decided that the employer was therefore not liable.

In *Best* v. *Staffordshire University*, the employer provided counselling as part of its occupational health services. However, the fact that the services were provided did not mean that there was any possibility in this particular case that the employer could or should have foreseen that Best would become ill.

In *Green* v. *Grimsby and Scunthorpe Newspapers Ltd*, the employee's complaint was that it took five days for the employer to respond to the employee's grievance about stress. This was not considered to be excessive, as had been alleged; rather, it was a reasonable length of time to enable a responsible employer to assess the correct approach to deal with the problem.

The employer's liability and the resulting award to the employee were upheld in *Moore* v. *Welwyn Components Ltd*. Here the employee complained of suffering depression caused by bullying at work. The employer was vicariously liable for the acts of the offending members of staff, but appealed the level of the award made against it on the grounds that external stress should have been taken into account as that was likely to cause him to become ill in the future in any case. That was rejected by the court as the employer had not provided evidence to show that there were any other causes that might have caused his illness and therefore be a future risk factor.

Occupational health perspective

Dealing with stress at work is a management problem, as can be seen above. Occupational health can play a role in supporting management when introducing and undertaking stress audits, developing relevant policies, and putting in place suitable stress awareness programmes. Unfortunately sometimes occupational health is called upon at too late a stage, perhaps when someone has become ill. At this point occupational health can advise management on a suitable return to work and rehabilitation programme and offer confidential support to the employee, particularly if there is access to professional counselling or an employee assistance programme. The two case studies presented below illustrate the disastrous health effects that stress at work can have on an individual. The case studies look at two different aspects of stress-related illness: the first is written from a client's personal perspective and demonstrates the potential outcome when there is a lack of control over work load and a poor level of management support, resulting in excessive demands upon a worker; the second is written from an occupational health perspective and serves to demonstrate not only the lack of a support element but also the effect of change and role identity. Both of these case studies relate to individuals who have spent several years in their chosen profession before succumbing to stress-related ill health.

Case study: a client's perspective

My working life started in 1974. I was a professionally qualified lawyer working in the public sector and by 2002 I had a legal team of 12 qualified staff and 12 non-legal staff.

The job was demanding and varied, with a large training element, provision of legal advice and liaison with the organisation's stakeholders. By 2002 I was aware that the demands of the role had expanded to such an extent that additional staff were required. In the drawing up of a business case to support the claim, it became clear that between 1997 and early 2003 there had been an increase in work amounting to 26%. The business case was supported by my line manager and the head of human resources who described it as a very good business case. But the request for additional

Cont.

staff was refused by the chief executive. The effects were felt immediately by me as I did not have the means to do the job. I knew that additional resources were required and that the staff reporting to me could not be pushed harder. I felt helpless, unable to assist those directly under my responsibility, and powerless to improve the situation, but I was still required to run this part of the organisation.

The long hours I worked increased in an attempt to make up the short fall. Alternative suggestions for a temporary post were refused. Over the five months following the refusal to address the case for increased help with more staff I developed physical symptoms of stress and anxiety, with weight loss, interrupted sleep, tearfulness both in the professional setting and privately, and a feeling of hopelessness.

By August 2003 I was medically unfit to work, and at the time of writing, November 2005, I remain a patient of a psychologist and psychiatrist, and unfit to work. The effects of prolonged work-related stress and ensuing ill health have caused me to lose confidence in myself and my abilities. The loss of concentration continues, making everyday living exhausting and unfocused. The anxiety caused by visiting places where former work colleagues may be seen leads to my having a pounding heart, nausea and fear. I had not been subject to mental illness in the past, and to lose your career in such circumstances is devastating. Should I be able to consider employment in time, I hazard to suggest my medical past makes me unemployable.

Case study: the occupational health perspective

Since leaving school Miss A had worked within a technical department of a public sector organisation. She began as a trainee and rose through the ranks over the next 20 years. She had studied at college and gained qualifications along the way. She was, in short, successful, confident and capable. Then she took a sideways move within the organisation, but the post was 'disestablished' and so she was redeployed within the same management division but to a different role from that for which she had been trained and qualified.

The duties of the new job were diverse. There was much to learn, and training was a big issue. She reflected on her previous role, where she had trained and gained experience over a period of years before being given the level of responsibility she was now expected to shoulder in the new job for which she had no training at all. It was as though she had been thrown in at the deep end and left to drown. Some of the emotions and symptoms she experienced included tiredness, headaches, irritability, lack of self-esteem, concentration, anxiousness and panic attacks. She felt she had lost control of her emotions, which ultimately led to clinical depression as a result of work related stress. She had to make numerous visits to a consultant psychiatrist as an outpatient and to a behavioural therapist who taught her cognitive behavioural therapy.

The hardest part of all was for her to admit that she was ill. Once she accepted she was ill, she felt she had a foundation on which she could build for the future. She had to relearn the most basic of skills, for example reading a book, writing reports, socialising, making new friends, trusting people again and having faith in her own abilities. By 2003 she was working in a new career, but still seeing her GP on a regular basis and still on medication. On occasions she still has to see the behavioural therapist and she says that each time she does she emerges as a stronger person. Miss A says that she considers herself lucky to have received the support and help of health care professionals to enable her to have made the recovery steps she has achieved.

References

1. Chartered Institute of Personnel and Development (2005) *Annual Sickness and Absence Survey*.
2. Confederation of British Industry (2004) *Room for Improvement: Absence and labour turnover 2004*.
3. http://www.hse.gov.uk/statistics/overall/ohsb0405.htm last accessed 29.11.05.
4. Royal College of Nursing (2004) *Confidentiality: RCN guidance for occupational health nurses*.
5. Faculty of Occupational Medicine (1999) *Guidance on Ethics for Occupational Physicians*.
6. Department for Work and Pensions (2004) *Building Capacity for Work: A UK framework for vocational rehabilitation*, Ref. ELCI 3.
7. Disability Discrimination Act 1995, part 2, paragraph 4.61. Code of Practice for the elimination of discrimination in the field of employment against disabled persons or persons who have a disability.
8. Waddell, G. & Burton, K. (2004) *Concepts of Rehabilitation for the Management of Common Health Problems*. TSO, London.
9. Pearson, A., Vaughan, B. (1986) *Nursing Models for Practice*. Heinemann, London.
10. www.who.int/classifications/icf/en last accessed 29.11.05.
11. Hughes, V. (ed.) (2004) *Tolley's Guide to Employee Rehabilitation*. Lexis Nexis Butterworths, London.
12. Leaflet E14, *What to do if your employee is sick*. HM Revenue & Customs.
13. Advisory, Conciliation and Arbitration Service (ACAS) *Absence and Labour Turnover and Health and Employment*. Advisory Booklet.
14. Health and Safety Executive (2000) *Securing Health Together*. HSE, London.
15. The Stationery Office (2002) *The Back Book: The Best Way to Deal with Back Pain*. TSO, London.
16. Judicial Studies Board (2004) *Guidelines for the Assessment of General Damages in Personal Injury Cases*, 7th edn. Oxford University Press, Oxford.
17. Health and Safety Executive (2005) *The Tiered System of Health Surveillance: brief guidance for employers and health professionals*. HSE, London.
18. Health and Safety Executive (2004) *The role of work stress and psychological factors in the development of musculo-skeletal disorders*. Research Report 273, Stress and MSD Study. HSE, London.
19. International Stress Management Association and ACAS in conjunction with the HSE (2004) *Working Together to Reduce Stress at Work: a guide for employees*.
20. Mackay, C. J., Cousins, R., Kelly, P. J., Lee, S. & McCaig, R. H. (2004) Management standards and work related stress in the UK: Policy background and science. *Work & Stress* (Apr–Jun) **18** (2), 91–112.
21. Health and Safety Executive (2004) *Management Standards for Tackling Work-Related Stress*. HSE, London.
22. *Barber* v. *Somerset Council* [2004] IRLR 475: the House of Lords clarified the requirements for stress claims to succeed.

Chapter 6
Termination of Employment

Employment law perspectives

It is unlawful to discriminate against a disabled worker by dismissing the person or subjecting them to any other detriment relating to their disability. This is a matter that must be borne in mind in the management of sickness absence, and particularly when the point is reached where termination of employment is a possible outcome. Properly managed, justified and with supporting evidence, the termination of employment through ill health retirement or dismissal can be fair, non-discriminatory and appropriate. Employers have to take account of their obligations under all of the employment legislation rules and standards. In this chapter we set out some of the main issues to consider in this respect.

Statutory procedures

The Employment Act 2002 (Dispute Resolution) Regulations were introduced in October 2004. They set the minimum legal standards to be followed in dismissal, disciplinary and grievance proceedings. Employers will be in breach of the Regulations if they do not follow them within their internal procedures. They include giving the employee the right to be accompanied (subject to the Regulations and the company policy) and to appeal the decision.

If an employer fails to follow these procedures this will make any resulting dismissal automatically unfair. Likewise an employee who claims constructive dismissal, or who wishes to pursue another type of tribunal claim against the employer, will be obliged first to have followed the proper internal procedures. Any compensation awarded as a result of a tribunal claim can be reduced or increased by between 10 and 50% to reflect a failure by either party to comply with the new rules. Full details of the Regulations and related guidance are available from the web sites: www.dti.gov.uk and www.businesslink.gov.uk.

The statutory dispute regulations, in summary, require a standard three-step procedure to be implemented when dismissal, including for disciplinary or capability-related reasons, or any early retirement terminations are addressed by the employer with the employee. The biggest change is that all forms of dismissal must be addressed in this way, including retirements such as in ill health situations and redundancies.

The steps are:

(1) The employer's written complaint, which must be sent to the employee so that he is informed of the basis of the dismissal or disciplinary hearing.

(2) The employer must arrange to meet the employee. The employee may be accompanied and is expected to take reasonable steps to attend. Where the result is not in favour of the employee, he must be informed of the decision and offered the right of appeal.

(3) An appeal hearing must be arranged by the employer. This should be conducted by a more senior manager than attended the meeting in Step 2, if this is practicable.

There is also a modified disciplinary and dismissal procedure, which is a two-step procedure and is to be used where summary dismissal has taken place on the grounds of gross misconduct, for example. The modified procedure steps are:

(1) The employer's letter setting out the reason for the dismissal and detailing the right of appeal.

(2) The appeal hearing as described above.

The employee is permitted, and in some cases (such as constructive dismissal) required by law, to take out a grievance, defined as 'a complaint by an employee about action which his employer has taken or is contemplating taking in relation to him' before bringing a claim in an employment tribunal. It is possible that an employee who is disgruntled about a procedure involving his return to work after sick leave or dissatisfied with other related matters could take out a grievance. Where a grievance is raised, the parties each have to follow the standard or modified steps as appropriate.

Sickness absence requires special consideration of procedural standards where there could be a risk for the employee of a dismissal on the grounds of incapability and/or the risk for the employer of inadvertent disability discrimination. It is worth remembering that, as covered in Chapter 5, the changes made to the Disability Discrimination Act mean that an employer usually cannot now use the justification defence for failing to make reasonable adjustments. The question for employers now is generally whether there are potential adjustments and whether those adjustments are reasonable or not.

Dismissal

The Employment Rights Act 1996 (ERA) provides that employees have the right not to be unfairly dismissed. The legislation sets out potentially fair reasons for dismissal. Those that relate to sickness, absence or long-term ill health dismissals usually cover one or more of the following reasons:

- *Conduct:* this is usually applicable to circumstances where there is no under-lying health reason for the absence, where there is frequent lateness or un-authorised absence, or where there is reasonable evidence to support the contention that an employee is malingering, or someone is otherwise not complying with company attendance and absence reporting standards. It can apply to frequent short-term absence situations, depending on the individual facts – for example, where an employee claims to be suffering from a hangover or other such excuse, this implies some responsibility on their part to choose to correct or improve their attendance. It is usual that an employer would be expected to take occupational health advice and go through the standard disciplinary verbal and written warnings process before effecting warnings or a dismissal in these situations.

- *Capability:* capability is a potentially fair reason for dismissal: ERA states that '. . . it is for the employer to show the reason for dismissal . . . [one reason is that the dismissal] relates to the capability or qualifications of the employee for performing work of the kind which he was employed by the employer to do'. Capability is usually a 'no blame' reason, which is applicable both to longer-term ill health absence and frequent short-term absence. These kinds of cases will relate to either frequent short-term or longer-term absence with an indication of an underlying medical cause, and, where the latter is identified as a factor, there is also no reasonable expectation of an improvement to attendance levels or a return to work is not possible in the foreseeable future. Before the decision to terminate the employment is taken, occupational health reports, a report from any treating specialist doctor and the patient's GP will be standard best practice requirements of the employer. Other expert reports may, where genuinely applicable, assist in the decision-making process – for example, a report from a psychologist in the case of an employee who has learning difficulties. The warnings process must be followed and full consideration of DDA requirements given, particularly with regard to reasonable adjustments and alternative employment considerations.

- *Some other substantial reason (SOSR):* this reason for dismissal can be used in its own right or as an additional reason combined with one or other of the foregoing reasons for dismissal. Where SOSR applies to the termination of employment decision, the substantial reason must be explained and it must be reasonable. In *Wilson* v. *Post Office* [2000] IRLR 834, for example, the Court of Appeal held that the employee had been dismissed for SOSR because his attendance record did not meet the required standard. Despite the absences being due to ill health, it was held that this was not a capability dismissal but one of SOSR.

- *Ill health retirement:* this is a term that is not actually a reason for dismissal as defined by ERA, the implication being that an ill health retirement is a situation where the employment is terminated by voluntary resignation and mutual agreement. If that is the case, the employment ends by consent and not dismissal. The usual train of events in these situations is that there will be an assessment and report of the individual's medical condition and this will recommend whether early retirement is supported. That report will be considered by the pension or insurance scheme administrators. The employer and employee must decide as a separate issue on the employment relationship's future. Clearly an ill health retirement cannot be effected unless and until the employment is ended. How it ends is the issue for management. If the employee agrees to resign, this is straightforward. If the employee does not wish to resign, the employer must make a decision based on the facts as he knows them and by following proper procedures. If the conclusion is to terminate the employment, there will be a dismissal in law usually based on both the 'capability' and 'SOSR' reasons combined. Following proper procedures must include those of statutory dispute procedures and DDA considerations.

- *Constructive dismissal* is a less usual situation whereby the employment relationship is terminated by the employee in circumstances involving some sort of dispute or grievance with the employer. Here the employee terminates the contract as a direct result of the employer's conduct. Examples of the kinds of situations where constructive dismissal can occur include 'whistle-blowing', harassment, and breach of statutory or contractual rights.

  In order to have a claim succeed on the grounds of constructive dismissal, an employee has to be able to show:
  ○ That there was a fundamental breach of the contract by the employer.
  ○ That this breach caused the employee to resign.
  ○ That the employee did not delay too long before resigning: this can be by leaving after a single incident has occurred of a sufficiently serious nature as to warrant the action, or by the 'final straw' incident of a series of incidents that culminate in the decision to leave.
  ○ That the employee used the appropriate internal dispute resolution procedure (grievance or appeal), or can show good reason not to have done so. It is usual in a constructive dismissal to consider the modified dispute procedures.

- *Frustration of contract* can sometimes, but comparatively rarely, apply to an ill health or poor attendance dismissal. Frustration of a contract implies that there is no fault on either party but that a situation exists whereby the contract cannot be performed in the future, and thus the contract is frustrated and its termination justified. The effect of this in legal reasoning is that the contract is then automatically deemed to have ended without a dismissal. However, caution and due regard to the particular case and individual circumstances will be necessary in these cases. Also, it may be prudent taking legal advice before any decision is made. Many employers who terminate an employment based on the doctrine of frustration will take the precaution of also effecting a dismissal on the grounds of incapacity.

Whatever the potentially fair reason for dismissal that an employer considers appropriate, an employment tribunal hearing the case, should the matter be challenged through litigation, is guided by ERA when making its decision having regard to:

'. . . the question of whether the dismissal was fair or unfair . . . depends on whether in the circumstances (including the size and resource of the employer's undertaking) the employer acted reasonably or unreasonably in treating it as a sufficient reason for dismissing the employee . . .'

Returning to the genuinely ill employee, it is essential to rely on the principles set out in the case of *East Lindsey District Council* v. *Daubney* [1977] IRLR 181 EAT, to which reference was made in Chapter 5, when dealing with these situations. The Daubney case demonstrated the requirement that the employee has to be given to understand that his continuing employment depends on his return to work. Rather than a disciplinary hearing, a meeting must be held with management that both complies with the statutory dispute procedures standards and also takes the form of a 'no blame' consultative meeting with the employee where he is warned of any risk to his employment. At the meeting, the prognosis of the medical condition, adjustments to the workplace, duties, etc. must be discussed with the employee.

What is fundamental is that, should there be no viable prospect of return, the employee must be given warnings that his job is at risk. Where there is no prospect of a return to work, the employer may have to look at terminating the employment with an ill health retirement. Suspending the employment, but leaving the employee 'on the books', may be appropriate when there is a permanent health insurance pay-out. If the ending of the employment is contemplated, the employer must give serious consideration to reasonable adjustments as required by the DDA. These could include a wide range of actions as exampled in more detail in Chapter 5.

At the point where termination of employment is reached, the employer must also consider alternative employment options. It is important to note a number of legal factors that come into play in these situations:

- An employee's contract of employment covers the terms and conditions for work on which they have been engaged. If there is a transfer to an alternative post, or a change in hours, or any other substantive change, then new contractual terms must be agreed by negotiation.
- Different permanent health insurance schemes (PHIs) provide a range of cover options and related terms and conditions. These should be consulted for the precise circumstances and provided to the employee. A PHI situation, whatever its outcome, does not obviate the need for the employer to follow proper procedures in the employment process in general. PHI is an insurance matter but it is not usually a matter over which the employer has control. In some PHI schemes the cover provides for qualification when an employee becomes permanently incapable, through ill health, of carrying out the duties for which they were employed. In these circumstances the employee may have entitlement to an award under the scheme and may go on to take up alternative employment.

  If an employee is entitled to an award under a PHI scheme, whatever its terms and conditions, the individual circumstances will need to be carefully considered. The fact that there is such an entitlement does not mean that the employer can base a dismissal decision on this rationale. The employment relationship is different from the insurance relationship. Some employers might argue that, where a PHI scheme provides a pay-out to the employee, the employer can take it as read that the employee is not able to return to work and the contract can be terminated and regarded as frustrated. This could prove to be unwise: there is an argument that a contract of employment that provides for PHI cover anticipates permanent ill health and that therefore frustration of contract is not applicable. There is also the question of compassion to be considered when employees are so ill that they cannot return to their work. Each case should be considered on its own facts and merits.

- How the employee will be notified and considered for any alternative posts is an important matter that needs to be planned and communicated properly. It is likely that occupational health assessments will be of great value in assisting with fitness evaluation for the alternative duties and any recommendations of adjustments. Consideration given to re-training and supervision will also be key parts of the proper process.

The onus is on the employer to keep in touch with the employee in all of these kinds of situations.

Medical and occupational health advice

It is for the employer and, if the case comes to court, the judiciary to make the decision as to whether the employee is deemed to be disabled within the meaning of the DDA. This is not a matter for the occupational health professional to decide, as we have mentioned previously. Rather, it is the medical or occupational health adviser's duty to provide the relevant information that will enable management, or the courts, to make their decisions. In order to allow the health professionals to provide their advice properly, the correct questions and information must be given by those making the enquiry. This does not necessarily mean that the employer needs to know the diagnosed medical condition. Although this can be helpful and pertinent in many cases, in others it can be withheld legitimately without compromising the advice on which the employer can choose to act.

The medical opinion and occupational health advice on the DDA factors should relate to the key qualifying factors of the Act (as detailed in Chapter 5) including, for example, addressing the questions of:

- Does the person have an impairment?
- Does this have an adverse effect on his ability to carry out normal day-to-day activities, such as:
  - mobility
  - manual dexterity
  - physical co-ordination
  - continence
  - ability to lift, carry or otherwise move everyday objects
  - speech, hearing or eyesight
  - memory or ability to concentrate, learn or understand
  - perception of the risk of physical danger
- Is the adverse effect substantial?
- Is the adverse effect long term or recurring?
- Can you provide examples of these effects and any work-related adjustments that might be appropriate for us to consider?

- Are these likely to be temporary or permanent?
- What review periods would be appropriate in these circumstances?

Unless there is a contractual obligation to a medical examination, an employer who insists on such an examination could be in breach of contract if they force the issue. Conversely, an employee who unreasonably refuses to undergo a medical examination risks the employer's being held to be legitimate in making its decisions based on the facts that are available.

Case law

The following cases show the importance of obtaining up-to-date medical reports and then taking due notice of the advice given, including the reasonable adjustment considerations. Both cases also appear to illustrate the need for line managers to be trained in dealing appropriately with these situations.

Spencer v. *O2 UK* (2004) ET Case No. 1805496/03 decision of 29 March 2004

Mr Spencer was diabetic. He was employed from February 1997 until his dismissal in September 2003. His attendance record was poor, with most absences being related to his medical condition, and some to do with his management of it and his medication. His employers began to take formal action about the absences in 2001. Between January and June 2003, he attended several consultation meetings. He was dismissed for SOSR – some other substantial reason. No up-to-date specialist report was obtained before the dismissal took place, with the last report being some 11 months old. The tribunal held that the decision to dismiss fell outside the band of reasonable responses and was therefore unfair. It was also disability discrimination by failing to take account of the fact that the employee's main problems occurred early in the morning. His working hours could have been considered for adjustment to a later start. Alternatively, part-time work could have been considered as an option. The case was then settled on terms agreed between the parties.

British Telecommunications plc v. *Pousson* [2004] EAT 0347/04

Mr Pousson worked in a call centre as a customer service adviser. He was a diabetic, which contributed to his suffering from occasional bouts of infection and minor illness. He was absent as a result at least four times over two years, which led to the BT performance attendance procedure being invoked. He felt under pressure to perform and he felt discouraged in leaving his desk to test his blood sugar levels as required. He suffered a hypoglycaemic attack and a head injury. He was absent from his job for two years and his employment was then terminated.

BT had referred Mr Pousson to its occupational health physician who had advised making adjustments to allow the employee time off duty to test his sugar levels and inject insulin, allowing him to access food and drink, and giving consideration to varying shift patterns to help him with control of his diabetes. The occupational health doctor also suggested that there was a link between the underlying diabetes and the viral infections and other minor illnesses suffered by Mr Pousson. The advice appears to have been largely not followed by management. The employee brought a claim of unlawful discrimination to an employment tribunal.

The tribunal found in favour of Mr Pousson and the decision was upheld by the Employment Appeal Tribunal. BT had not implemented the reasonable adjustments as advised, nor had they provided their managers with the necessary guidance or training to deal with employees who have a disability.

Archibald v. *Fife Council* [2004] IRLR 651

This case dealt with the question of reasonable adjustment in the sense of offering suitable alternative employment. A disabled employee became unfit to do the manual work of a road-sweeper for which she had been employed before suffering a back injury. She became fit to work only in a sedentary occupation and she was found to be disabled within the meaning of the Disability Discrimination Act 1995. It was discriminatory on the part of the employer to require her to compete with a non-disabled person for a clerical job. The case decision indicates that where an employee becomes disabled, or where the existing disability worsens, and no suitable adjustment would make them fit to do the work they did before, consideration must be given to a transfer to a suitable alternative post if one is available. The employee should not be put to a disadvantage in making their application for such a transfer.

Taylorplan Catering (Scotland) Ltd v. *McInally* [1980] IRLR 53

Mr McInally was employed as a barman on a recreation facility for oil-rig workers. He worked alone and was required to be of a strong disposition and healthy as there was no back-up for him. His dismissal for his frequent absence was fair because the company could not run this important facility without his regular attendance at work. Even if one illness did not recur, there were others that had cropped up so regularly that he could not be relied on to have a clean bill health for any substantial period of time.

This case examples the issue of considering the likelihood of an illness recurring or some other illness arising, balanced against the business needs of the employer. The length of the various absences and the spaces of good health between them would be important to consider in these cases. This would also help to establish whether there was a pattern and whether absences or presences are consistent. Employers in most sectors would also need to consider recommendations to vary hours or otherwise make adjustments to enable employees to recover working health and reach required reliability standards.

Employment tribunals

Despite every effort, some cases will lead to the doors of the courts. In relation to matters concerning employment disputes, employers and employees are now required first to use internal procedures, before taking legal action.

The Employment Tribunals were created in 1964, originally to hear appeals against certain expenses imposed by statutory bodies during industrial training. Their functions rapidly grew, and the aim was to provide fast, inexpensive and informal access to justice in disputes about employment. They were called industrial tribunals for many years but are now known as employment tribunals, and they have a much wider remit today. The number of cases, and their often complex nature, means that the tribunals now are a long way from the original aims in some respects. While the relative informality of proceedings and the right to self-represent continues today, some form of representation is becoming more prevalent now, given the complexity of employment legislation and case law.

At the tribunal, witnesses give evidence on oath or affirmation but all parties usually remain seated during the course of the proceedings, and there are no wigs and gowns. The tribunals are courts and each panel is made up of a chairman, who is a solicitor or a barrister with suitable experience and qualifications, and two lay members with respective experience from management and staff sides of industry.

The main jurisdiction of the employment tribunals is in connection with employment disputes arising out of allegations by an individual applicant, the Claimant, against his employer, the Respondent. The Claimant may be an employee, but others such as temporary workers have the right to bring complaints under discrimination law and breaches of regulations. They also may challenge the employment status claimed by the agency or the end user of their services, and so have unfair dismissal and related claims rights in the tribunals.

Many complaints do not require a qualifying period of employment to gain the right to come under the jurisdiction of the tribunals, but unfair dismissal claims, for example, can only be brought by people who have at least one year's qualifying service. Alleged acts of discrimination or breaches of statutory rights give rise to an instant qualification to bring a complaint before the tribunal. Employees must also follow guidelines by bringing their complaint within certain deadlines and by doing so in the proper manner. Employers are required to respond properly and within specified deadlines if they wish to defend the claim. Full details and updates can be obtained from the tribunals' website: www.employmenttribunals.gov.uk.

It is worth visiting a tribunal as an observer to watch and learn from the experience before perhaps attending to give evidence in a case. Most tribunals are open to the public. It is courteous to arrive before the start time of that particular tribunal office – usually the start time is between 9.30 a.m. and 10.00 a.m., but this can vary – and to explain to the clerk why you are there.

The employment tribunals' website gives current guidance as to the conduct, and general information including details of what happens at hearings, forms, deadlines, etc. These details should be checked regularly as there are changes made on a fairly frequent basis.

With regard to advice on the tribunal case itself, how to manage it and handle pleadings and communications in cases that have not settled, there are many specialists who provide employment law advice for which charges are made to the client. There are also voluntary organisations that can offer assistance, such as the Citizens Advice Bureau and the Free Representation Unit.

Occupational health personnel are liable to be involved in matters relating to the termination of employment for health-related reasons and could therefore be called to give evidence. They may be required to attend as witnesses to give evidence about other employment dispute matters, such as in absence management, disability related discrimination cases, or health and safety cases.

Increasingly, nurses and doctors are witness to fact – saying what actually happened – and/or as experts giving an opinion as to whether procedures were adequate. In the latter instance in, for example, a disability discrimination claim, the tribunal may need to hear why a person was considered unfit to do a particular job and why reasonable adjustments could not have been made from the medical point of view.

The expert witness

If occupational health professionals are called as expert witnesses at a court or tribunal, it is important that they know that they are under a duty to give opinions according to their specific expertise, not merely to state observed facts. Such opinions will assist the achievement of the overriding objective of a fair disposal of the case under consideration.

The courts require that the expert witness is not there to represent the interests of the instructing party. Rather, the duty is to the interests of justice as a whole. In many cases, each party will instruct his own expert, unless agreement can be reached. There is a tendency towards the appointment of a single joint expert who is either appointed by agreement between the parties or imposed by the tribunal, leaving the embattled opponents to consider whether there is any valid reason for them to bring their own expert in to raise any points of dispute. It is recommended that those who may be required to give evidence as an expert witness attend a suitable training programme. The Expert Witness Institute has a Code of Guidance, which can be found at www.ewi.org.uk./code_of_guidance.asp.

Advisory, Conciliation and Arbitration Service (ACAS)

ACAS provides an excellent conciliation service to both sides involved in tribunal cases, and can offer impartial and independent advice that may help to settle such cases. In conciliated settlements, both the parties, Claimant and Respondent, need to reach a compromise agreement between them that is assisted by the ACAS conciliation service.

There is also the arbitration service now offered by ACAS, which provides a voluntary alternative to the employment tribunal for the resolution of unfair dismissal disputes in the form of arbitration. Resolution of disputes under the ACAS Arbitration Scheme[1] is intended to be confidential, informal, relatively fast and cost-efficient. Procedures under the Scheme are non-legalistic, and far more flexible than the traditional model of the employment tribunal and the courts. For example, the Scheme avoids the use of formal pleadings and formal witness and documentary procedures. Strict rules of evidence will not apply, and as far as possible, instead of applying strict law or legal precedent, general principles of fairness and good conduct will be taken into account (including, for example, principles referred to in any relevant ACAS 'Disciplinary and Grievance Procedures' code of practice or 'Discipline at Work' handbook). Arbitral decisions ('awards') will be final, with very limited opportunities for parties to appeal or otherwise challenge the result.

Age discrimination

Regulations have been published by government in order to provide the necessary legislation to prevent discrimination on the grounds of age.[2] The UK had to comply with the requirement to implement the *Framework Directive for Equal Treatment in Employment and Occupation* (2000/78/EC) by October 2006. Case law on age discrimination will initially look to the now well established precedents and examples provided by other types of discrimination cases. The potential developments of age discrimination law will continue as legal challenges take place when the laws and related regulations take effect.

There are various sources of reliable advice available at no cost to employers preparing to meet the challenges and opportunities that will come from the age discrimination legislation: for example, www.acas.org.uk and www.dti.gov.uk.

Age discrimination laws protect all age groups from acts of discrimination or harassment within employment. This extends to occupational health related policies and practices. Any employment protocols must apply equally and/or have an objective reason for any actions that treat one group of workers differently from another. It will be a matter of added value to employers to address policy procedure reviews using the expertise of occupational health practitioners, particularly with reference to age-related change issues.

A useful summary of the main provisions of the legislation and a checklist for employers is provided on the website at www.agepositive.gov.uk. Included in the information is the following guidance and FAQS.

The practical implications of the right not to be discriminated against on the grounds of age will impact upon the employment processes of recruitment,

---

Age Positive Guidance and FAQ

Ten key points

(1) The Employment Equality (Age) Regulations are in force from 1 October 2006.

(2) Regulations cover employment and vocational training. This includes access to career guidance, recruitment advice, promotion, development, termination, perks and pay.

(3) The regulations cover people of all ages, both old and young.

(4) All employers, providers of vocational training, trade unions, professional associations, employer organisations and trustees, and managers of occupational pension schemes will have new obligations to consider.

(5) Goods, facilities and services are not included in these regulations.

(6) Upper age limits for unfair dismissal and redundancy will be removed.

(7) A national default retirement age of 65 will be introduced, making compulsory retirement below age 65 unlawful (unless objectively justified). This will be reviewed in 2011.

(8) All employees will have the 'right to request' to work beyond the default retirement age of 65 or any other retirement age set by the company, and all employers will have a 'duty to consider' requests from employees to work beyond 65.

(9) Occupational pensions are covered by the regulations, as are employer contributions to personal pensions. However, the regulations generally allow pension schemes to work as they do now. See regulations for more details.

(10) The regulations do not affect state pensions.

Answers to ten questions

(1) Who does the law cover?
- All workers including the self-employed, contract workers, office holders, the police and members of trade organisations.
- People who apply for work and, in some instances, people who have left work.
- People taking part in or applying for employment-related vocational training, including all courses at Further Education and Higher Education institutions.

(2) Who isn't covered by the regulations?
- Members of the regular armed forces, full-time and part-time reservists.
- Unpaid volunteers.

(3) What does vocational training cover?
- All forms of training and retraining courses, practical work experience and guidance that contributes to employability, training provided by employers or private and voluntary sector providers, vocational training provided by further and higher education institutions and adult education programmes.

(4) What do the regulations cover?
- Direct and indirect discrimination, harassment and victimisation. Employers can be held responsible for the actions of employees in all four cases.

(5) Are there any circumstances in which treatment on grounds of age will be lawful?
- Exemptions will be allowed on Genuine Occupational Requirement (GOR) and if there is an objective justification. However, both are likely to be difficult to prove.
- The 'test of objective justification' means employers will have to show, with evidence, that they are pursuing a legitimate aim and that it is an appropriate and necessary (proportionate) means of achieving that aim.
- The legislation will protect individuals or companies who are forced to discriminate on age grounds in order to comply with other legislation, e.g. bar staff serving alcohol must be at least 18.

(6) My employees' pay and benefits vary according to length of service. Can this continue?
- Benefits based on a length of service requirement of five years or less – the 'five year exemption' – will be exempted and will be able to continue.
- After the five-year exemption, employers must show that there will be an advantage from rewarding loyalty, encouraging the motivation or recognising the experience of workers by awarding benefits on the basis of length of service.

(7) How does the legislation impact on the national minimum wage?
- Employers will be able to follow the age bands and minimum wage levels used in the national minimum wage legislation.

(8) What should I know about the default retirement age?
- The default retirement age will be set at 65 for both men and women. It means mandatory retirement before that age will be unlawful unless a lower age can be exceptionally objectively justified. It does not mean you need to

Cont.

set a retirement age at 65 either – you can operate with no retirement age, or set a retirement age of 65 or higher. All employees will have the 'right to request' to work beyond any retirement age.

- Employers will have new time-bound responsibilities to inform employees of their 'right to request' and they will have a 'duty to consider' all such applications.
- Where an extension of work is agreed, the 'right to request' and 'duty to consider' will remain in place when retirement is next considered.

(9) What will the new regulations say about occupational pension schemes?

- Occupational pension schemes are included (although the draft legislation allows occupational pension schemes in general to work as they do at present).
- Personal pensions not provided by the employer (except the employer's own contribution) are not covered by the draft regulations.
- Employers will be able to provide different pension schemes to employees of different ages or with different lengths of service, and use minimum and maximum ages for admission to pension schemes and for the payment of pensions.
- The details are fully outlined in the Draft Regulations – see how to access these below.

(10) What should I do now?

- Review your employment policies and practices.
- Seek advice if you have concerns. If you do not have access to your own legal advice, ACAS is the nominated agency to give advice and guidance on age issues.
- Be Prepared.

These key facts and answers are for information only as provided by the DTI.[3]

training, career development and termination of employment, including retirement and dismissal. Workplace policies and procedures will be reviewed and revised to 'age-proof' these and effect the necessary compliance. Eradicating ageism will be challenging: as with other forms of anti-discrimination, cultural change at work will be as important as establishing the policies and practice.

There is no doubt that age discrimination has existed, and this is evident in the thinking and expression of values that have been exhibited up to the point of being made unlawful. They exist in the everyday workplace culture and in the formal communications of the employer in advertisements, policies, etc. For example, most people will have heard the phrase 'he's past his sell-by date' used at work, or 'she's just a kid, she can't do that job at her age'. And then there are the birthday cards, such as those that have the general 'over the hill' or 'past it' message often combined with a picture to further illustrate the point of seeming decrepitude with advancing years.

Many job advertisements have in the recent past been openly specific about the age range that is welcome to apply; others have not used a number to send out the message but have made it clear that they are just as specific by their choice of language, using words such as, mature, young, experienced or newly qualified. In the everyday situation at work, evidence of harassment or discrimination may also be prevalent. This could include opportunities for training and promotion or transfers not being considered on an equal basis because of age.

There are also implications for the occupational health professions that arise from age discrimination legislation, probably more than from many other aspects of anti-discrimination law. Currently, employment legislation exists to protect young people at work from the health and safety perspective: for example, restricted hours of work under working time regulations. Despite a predicted older workforce this trend has not as yet been considered for any particular risk assessment need. As far as health assessments are concerned, the regulations indicate that it will be justifiable to carry out a medical test in order to ensure that an individual is fit to do the job required.[4] It also appears to be the case that it will not be direct discrimination to require medical examinations for appointment to a position, continuing in post, or promotion where there are health requirements that apply to all persons in such positions regardless of their age. It may be indirect discrimination, however, to carry out medical tests on employees if those in a particular age group are less likely to pass the test than others in a different age group. But there are exemptions and exceptions in the Age Regulations which include:

- Pay related to the National Minimum Wage
- Enhanced redundancy payments
- Life assurance
- Acts under statutory authority

It is the last point which is of particular importance to occupational health. Age criteria are used in legislation that covers various licences and health clearances for certain jobs. Where this is the case it continues to be lawful, and indeed the employer must continue, to follow those criteria as laid down by statute. Employers will not be acting in contravention of age discrimination regulations by following their statutory duty as prescribed by the relevant body, for example, DVLA, CAA etc. It will be worth checking regularly for changes to those statutory requirements, as is always the case, but unless or until these are modified they must be followed.

It is unlawful to make assumptions on ability or capability to a job based solely on age. Where an employer does consider that age and health-related factors are an issue, the Chartered Institute of Personnel and Development recommends consultation with an occupational health or medical practitioner (see www.cipd.co.uk). Flexible working is a feature of younger workers with family commitments and of disabled employees or those returning after an illness. This is likely to become a feature for older workers nearing the traditional retirement stage of their career. The CIPD's research in 2005 indicated that older workers, too, would welcome the chance to work flexibly or in altered working arrangements, part time, working from home, etc. in order to extend their employment beyond the retirement age and perhaps towards a phased retirement plan.

In redundancy situations, the length of service is to be retained as part of the statutory redundancy calculation rules, along with the age bands and multipliers within the formula. The maximum length of service is to remain set at 20 years and likewise the qualifying service is to remain at 2 years or more. The statutory redundancy rules are changed to take account of the Age Regulations, by removal of the lower age limit to qualify (it was age 18), and removal of the upper age limit and tapering formula which excluded or reduced payments to persons aged over 65.

Further practical information can be found in the ACAS guide for employers, *Age and the Workplace: Putting the Employment Equality (Age) Regulations 2006 into Practice*, which was published in April 2006.

Occupational health perspectives

For many people, the end of their employment will pass by without reference to the occupational health service. If the company provides advice on retirement then occupational health may help by giving health and health resources information as part of health promotion and health education. However, occupational health professional expertise is required when there are health aspects related to the termination of employment.

Occupational health may be asked to decide whether a person is:

- Fit to do the job.
- Fit to do the job with reasonable adaptations or adjustments.
- Not fit to do the job.

This may seem simple, but the occupational health professional will have to make recommendations based on the information given which will, or should, include:

- Referral letter from the line manager or human resources, depending on company policy – see Appendix 4 for an example.
- Sickness absence history.
- Job description.
- Job risk assessment.
- Hours of work.
- Location.
- Home address and travel arrangements.

As noted previously, by providing their report the occupational health services should not breach confidentiality by giving the manager or human resources the actual diagnosis and medical condition provided the employee gives express permission for this (see Appendix 7). Sometimes the prognosis and any adjustment or adaptation recommendations will be provided instead.

It is wise in most cases for occupational health to encourage the employee to talk to his manager and explain the situation with regard to his medical condition as far as possible. But there will be situations – such as with bullying, harassment or stress-related illness – where this may not be possible, and disclosure is not appropriate or could make matters even worse. It may be that the employee would prefer to give written permission for the occupational health doctor or nurse to speak to the manager on his behalf. Occupational health may also be asked to decide whether 'this person will come under the DDA'. This is not a decision for occupational health to make, but they do need to give sufficient, relevant information, based on the health assessment, to enable management to make an appropriate decision (see Appendix 8).

At the health assessment, it may help occupational health to consider the five steps of disability analysis. This is particularly relevant where adaptations may be necessary or consideration of the key factors under the DDA comes into play. The five steps to disability analysis are:

- *Functional history:* considering what the individual is capable of and not what they are incapable of – in other words, taking a positive approach.
- *Observations:* what you can see they are capable of doing.
- *Examination:* physical examination where necessary and indicated.
- *Logical reasoning of evidence:* considering all available evidence, including GP and specialist opinions where necessary.
- *Justification of opinions:* based on the evidence of all above.

For occupational health nurses, it may also be useful to consider the 'activities of daily living' as described by Roper *et al.*[5] and on which their model of nursing is based. These are:

- maintaining a safe environment
- communicating
- breathing
- eating and drinking
- eliminating
- personal cleansing and dressing
- controlling body temperature
- mobilising
- working and playing
- expressing sexuality
- sleeping
- dying

When at work the employee should be able to maintain maximum independence on the majority of these activities, and consideration should be given as to what adaptations or adjustments may be needed to help maintain that independence. Even those activities which do not appear to be relevant in a work situation need to be considered; these include expressing sexuality if there have been hormonal changes following therapeutic interventions and the ability to deal with personal cleansing and dressing in certain industries such as catering or laboratories handling hazardous compounds or organisms. Help can be sought for employment purposes from many of the specialist organisations, such as the Royal National Institute for the Blind, Job Centre Plus and the various illness support charities and government agencies. For example, 'Access to Work' is available from Job Centre Plus and sets out to help people overcome the problems resulting from disability. Job Centre Plus offers practical advice and help in a flexible way that can be tailored to suit the needs of an individual in a particular job. As well as giving advice and information to disabled people and employers, it is able to provide grants towards any extra employment costs that result from a person's disability.

For those facing redundancy, occupational health may be able to arrange for confidential support through counselling services or employee assistance programmes (EAPs) to help allay fears and anxieties at a difficult time. In this way, occupational health can make a positive contribution to the continued employment for both the employer and employee, or help to ease the way into retirement, ill health retirement or redundancy.

The legislation on age discrimination will have an impact on the work of the occupational health service. There are subjective values that exist about age and health status, such as older workers having less physical strength and endurance, or reduced cognitive capacity compared with younger people. A recent HSE research report deals with these, and many other misconceptions about age from an evidence-based perspective. [6] It may be wise to read research reports and act upon empirical data findings, particularly in the light of developing case law and legislative changes related to age discrimination.

References

1. ACAS Arbitration Scheme (England and Wales) Order 2001 SI No. 1185.
2. Employment Equality (Age) Regulations 2006.
3. Department of Trade and Industry (2005) *Age Positive: Tackling age discrimination and promoting age diversity in employment*. www.agepositive.gov.uk
4. Department of Trade and Industry. *Equality and Diversity: Coming of age*. DTI Employment Equality (Age) Regulations 2006 (in draft).
5. Roper, N., Logan, W., Tierney, A. (1980) *The Elements of Nursing*. Churchill Livingstone, Edinburgh.
6. Health and Safety Executive (2005) *Facts and misconceptions about age, health status and employability*. HSL/2005/20.

Appendix 1
Occupational Health Service Confidentiality Policy

The provision of a confidential, informed and impartial service to the individuals, departments, and external organisations that use the occupational health service (OHS) is essential in order to maintain a professional relationship of trust with them.

It is incumbent on all the staff of the OHS to maintain confidentiality. Each member of staff has an obligation not to divulge any information learned in respect of his or her work activities within the OHS, as detailed in the form below.

---

1. Clinical staff

Information about an individual may be disclosed to a third party outside the OHS only if:

- The individual him/herself has given informed and express consent for this in writing.
- You are required to give such information by a court of law.
- Disclosure is in the public interest.
- Agreed disclosure is for the purposes of medical research approved by an ethics committee.

2. Administrative staff

Any matter relating to patients of the OHS, including personal details, health or medical information, including diagnosis, investigation, or treatment, and advice sought and/or given, whether from patients' records or from other sources, must not be divulged to any third party by administrative staff *without exception*.

All such enquiries about an individual, or individuals, whether from a third person or from the individual personally, *must* be referred to a clinical member of staff.

No medical or health advice, information, recommendation or opinion is to be given by administrative staff *without exception*. All enquiries about health or medical matters must be referred to a clinical member of staff.

3. Any breaches of the above may result in disciplinary action, including dismissal.

I agree not to disclose any confidential information about patients or clients as described above.

Signature: ....

Date: ....

Appendix 2
Sample Pre-employment Health Assessment Form

Reproduced by kind permission of Dr Stuart Whitaker. Published by the Department of Health (1998) *The Management of Health, Safety and Welfare Issues for NHS Staff*. Crown copyright.

To be completed by the appointing officer

I would like to request that a pre-employment health assessment be undertaken for the purpose of safe job placement for the following applicant.

Applicant's name: . . . .
Job title: . . . .
Department: . . . .   Start date: --/--/----
Hours of work: Full time [ ]   If part time give hours: . . . .

Enclosed   Current job description   [ ]
             Applicant's employment history   [ ]
             Applicant's sickness absence record   [ ]

Signature: Date: --/--/----
Appointing officer:
Contact number:

To be completed by the applicant
Please read this form all the way through before starting to complete it

The purpose of pre-employment health assessment is to ensure, so far as is possible, that you are fit for the post you have applied for in order to protect your own and others' health and safety.

Questions are asked about your past and present health, medical treatment and any impairments that may have implications for health and safety. The information you provide will remain confidential to the occupational health department.

If you have any difficulties completing this form or wish to discuss any issues in a confidential setting, please contact the occupational health department for advice.

Declaration

I declare that all of the following statements and information is true to the best of my knowledge.

Signed: . . . .   Date: --/--/----

Personal details

Last name: . . . .

First names: . . . .

Sex: Male [ ] Female [ ]   Date of birth: --/--/----

Address: . . . .

. . . .

Postcode: . . . .

Telephone number: . . . .

Name and address of your general practitioner/family doctor: . . . .

. . . .

Postcode: . . . .

Vaccination history

Have you ever had any of the following vaccinations or tests? Please indicate YES, NO or Don't know. Please give dates and test results where known.

Immunisation	YES	NO	Don't know	Dates	Date of test result
Tetanus					
Poliomyelitis					
Rubella (German measles)					
TB test (Heaf, Tine, Mantoux)					
BCG (TB vaccination)					
Diphtheria					
Hepatitis A					
Hepatitis B Injection No. 1 Injection No. 2 Injection No. 3 Blood test Booster dose Blood test					

Please answer all of the following questions. If you answer **YES** please give details in the space provided on the back of this form.

		YES	NO	Don't know
1	Do you have any impairment that may affect your ability to work safely?			
2	Do you have any eyesight problems not corrected with glasses?			
3	Do you have any hearing problems not corrected with a hearing aid?			
4	Do you have any difficulty in standing, bending, lifting or other movements?			
5	Have you seen a doctor in the last year for any kind of health problem?			
6	Are you having any treatment or investigations of any kind at the moment?			
7	Are you waiting for any treatment or investigation?			
8	Have you ever had any kind of skin problem?			
9	Have you ever had any kind of back problem?			
10	Have you ever had any kind of problem with your joints including pain, swelling or stiffness?			
11	Have you ever had any mental illness or psychological problems?			
12	Have you ever had a drug or alcohol problem?			
13	Have you ever had fits, blackouts or epilepsy?			
14	Do you have any allergies?			
15	Have you ever had asthma, bronchitis or chest problems?			
16	Have you ever had treatment for tuberculosis (TB)?			
17	In the last 12 months have you had a cough for more than 3 weeks, ever coughed up blood or had any unexplained loss of weight or fever?			
18	Have you ever had hepatitis or jaundice?			
19	Have you ever had diabetes, or thyroid or gland problems?			
20	Do you have any other medical conditions?			
21	Have you ever had any illness that may have been caused or made worse by your work?			

What is your height?. . . . . What is your weight?. . . . .

In this section please give details of any of the questions to which you have answered **YES**. Details that may be useful include:

(a) How long did you have this problem for?
(b) When was this?
(c) What type of treatment, if any, did you receive?
(d) Were you admitted to hospital, unable to work or prevented from carrying out your normal activities because of the problem?
(e) Does the condition continue to affect you in any way?

Question number	Details

Please continue on a separate sheet of paper if necessary.

Appendix 3
COSHH Surveillance Registration Form

This form (HS1) is to be completed by the area safety officer if a COSHH assessment indicates health surveillance is necessary for an individual potentially exposed to hazardous substances. All such individuals must be registered for health surveillance with the occupational health service **BEFORE** work is commenced.

Is this registration in accordance with a current valid COSHH assessment?	Yes/No

Details of person to be registered

Surname:	Forenames:	M/F
Job title:	Date of birth:	
Department:	Place of work:	
Contact telephone number:		

Hazardous substance(s):	Details of exposure(s): e.g. frequency, duration, intensity
1.	
2.	
3.	

Personal protective equipment (PPE)/Respiratory protective equipment (RPE). If worn, what type?

Signature: . . . .   Date: . . . .
Print name: . . . .

Please return the form to:
For office use only:

Type of surveillance required:

Appendix 4
Management Referral Letter

TO: OCCUPATIONAL HEALTH DEPARTMENT

Date: .... From: ....

Please can you arrange to see the following employee, who has been advised of this referral and its purpose?

Personal details

Name: .... Date of birth: ....

Address: ....

....

.... Postcode: .... Tel no: ....

Employment details

Job title: .... Dept: .... Shift: ....

Manager: ....

Reason for referral (please tick ☑):

☐ Changing job requirements
☐ Following sickness absence
☐ Following accident or incident at work
☐ Other reason (please state): ....

....

Sick absence details for the past 12 months (longer if appropriate):

From	To	Reason given for absence

Information required from this referral (please tick ☑):

☐ **1.** Is he/she fit to carry out the full range of duties relating to his/her job?
☐ **2.** Will he/she be able to offer a regular and efficient service?
   3. If he/she is not fit at present for his/her full range of duties, please advise on:
☐   (a) Probable date of fitness to resume normal duties.
☐   (b) Whether restricted duties are required to facilitate a return to work as part of a rehabilitation programme. If so please give details.
☐ **4.** If he/she is permanently unfit for his/her present position, please comment on:
☐   (a) Whether re-deployment would allow a return to work.
☐   (b) If a return to work were not possible, would you support an application for retirement on the grounds of ill health?
☐ **5.** Other adjustments advised on health grounds: ....

....

Description and requirements of job process (please tick ☑):

- ☐ Bending/stooping
- ☐ Twisting of upper body
- ☐ Twisting of neck
- ☐ Arms at/above shoulder height
- ☐ Work with arms outstretched
- ☐ Forcible arm movements
- ☐ Rotation/twisting of forearm
- ☐ Forcible hand/wrist movements
- ☐ Forcible gripping movements
- ☐ Wrist repetition/wrist movements
- ☐ Use of hand/wrist at awkward angles
- ☐ Repetitive use of manual screwdriver
- ☐ Pincer grip movements

- ☐ Foot/leg movements
- ☐ Prolonged standing
- ☐ Working at heights
- ☐ Use of display screen equipment
- ☐ Use of vibrating tools
- ☐ Food handling
- ☐ FLT driving
- ☐ Contact with respiratory sensitisers/irritants
- ☐ Contact with dermatological sensitisers/ irritants
- ☐ Working at heights/confined spaces
- ☐ Other

Additional information:

. . . .

. . . .

The reason for this referral has been explained by:

Name: . . . . Signature: . . . . Date: . . . .

I confirm that the reasons regarding this referral have been discussed with me and I consent to a report being prepared by the occupational health department in relation to this referral. I accept that information relating to this referral will be held under the rules governing Medical Confidentiality and the Data Protection Act.

Employee's signature: . . . . Date: . . . .

Appendix 5
Letter to Employee Requesting Attendance at Occupational Health

Date

Dear [*name of employee*],

Re: Yourself and [*name of employer*]

We are sorry to learn that you continue to be unwell and look forward to exploring ways to help you recover your health and seeing you back at work.

You have now been off sick since [*enter date*], and according to company policy we would like you to attend the occupational health department for a consultation with [*enter name and designation*]. The purpose of the meeting will be to discuss your health and the best way forward for you to return to work. Please ring the occupational health department on [*insert phone number*] to make a mutually convenient appointment.

We wish you well and look forward to hearing from you soon. If you have any queries or concerns please do not hesitate to contact us.

Yours sincerely,

[*Add name and designation*]

Appendix 6
Letter to GP or Specialist Requesting Information

Date

Dear

Re: [*name of client/patient, address and date of birth*]

Your above named patient, who works for our organisation, has given his/her consent for us to obtain a medical report from you in order that we can make an assessment of his/her fitness to work. We enclose a copy of his/her consent, and a job description is also enclosed for your information.

The absence record is summarised as follows:
* Total days lost: . . . .
* Days lost this month: . . . .
* Days lost in previous months: . . . .

Can you please advise on the following? (*delete or amend as applicable*)
* How long is this episode of absence likely to last?
* Is there any underlying medical reason for this attendance record?
* Is he/she likely to render regular and efficient service in the future?
* What is the likely date of return to work?
* Will there be any disability at that time?
* Are there any reasonable adjustments we could make to accommodate the disability?
* Is there any specific recommendation you wish to make about him/her that would help in finding him/her an alternative job?

I would be grateful for an early reply and enclose a stamped addressed envelope.

Yours sincerely,

[*Add name and designation*]

Appendix 7
Employee Consent for Disclosure

I [*insert name*] of [*insert address*] hereby consent to the occupational health service giving:

(a) Details of my medical condition
(b) Access to my medical records

(*Delete as appropriate*)

To: [*insert name of organisation and/or department*]

I have been informed of my rights under the Access to Medical Reports Act 1988.

*I wish to have access to the report first.

*I am happy to see the report after it is supplied to [*insert name of organisation and/or department*]

*I do not wish to see the report.

(*Delete as appropriate*)

Signed: . . . .
Date: . . . .

Appendix 8
Report Form to Management

Confidential

Date: . . . .

To: . . . .

Re: [*Insert employee's name, job title and department*]

Thank you for asking occupational health to see [*insert name*]. I am now able to inform you that:

[*Delete as appropriate*]

- He/she is fit to carry out the full range of normal duties relating to his/her job
- He/she is/will be able to offer regular and efficient service
- He/she will probably be able to return to normal duties on (*give date*)
- He/she will be able to return to work subject to the following adjustments:

[*Insert adjustments advice*]

- He/she is unfit to return to this post and would benefit from redeployment
- He/she is unfit to return to this post and we would support an application for retirement on ill health grounds
- [*Other – insert as appropriate*]

Signed: . . . . Designation: . . . .

Date: . . . .

Appendix 9

Medical Records and Report Consent Form

To: ....

Date: ....

On behalf of: ....

I wish to obtain medical records and a report from [*insert name of doctor/specialist*] for the following purposes:

(1) to ascertain the prospect of your return to work;

(2) to ascertain any reasonable adjustments to your workload or system of work to facilitate your resumption of the duties for which you are employed.

Authorising signature: .... Designation: ....

Employee rights under the Access to Medical Reports Act 1988

1. You can ask to see the medical records and report before the company receives it. This request for access can be made either:
    (a) to the company when you grant us permission to obtain it (in which case we will tell the doctor of your request, and let you know when we apply);
    or
    (b) direct to the doctor at a later date, but before the records and report are supplied to the company.
2. If you ask to see the records and report:
    (a) you must contact the doctor to arrange access within 21 days of the company applying for the report, otherwise the doctor can give the records and report to us without showing them to you and without your consent (under 1(b) above you must contact the doctor within 21 days of notifying that you wish to see the records and report);
    (b) having seen the records and report, you can ask the doctor (in writing) to amend anything that you think is incorrect or misleading. If the doctor does not agree, a statement of your views will be attached;
    (c) provided you have seen them, the records and report will not be given to us unless you give the doctor your consent.
3. You will not be entitled to see any part of the records or report which:
    (a) the doctor believes could seriously harm your physical or mental health, or that of others;
    (b) indicates the doctor's intentions in respect of you;
    (c) reveals information about another person, or the identity of someone who has given the doctor information about you (unless that person consents or is a health professional involved in your care).
4. The doctor will tell you why access to the whole or part of the records or report is refused. Your rights of amendment will apply only to the disclosed part of the records or report. The doctor will only give the records and the report to the company with your consent.
5. You do not have to give the company permission to obtain medical information. (However, the inability to obtain up-to-date medical information may affect decisions made about your employment with the company.)
6. You may ask to see any medical information relating to you that the doctor has provided for employment purposes in the last six months (if prepared on or after 1.1.89). Such a request should be made to your doctor.

Appendix 10
Stress Risk Assessment Example Template

This table lists some examples of action planning to reduce the risk of work-related stress problems.

Stress risk assessment
• Identify the hazards • Decide who might be harmed and how • Assess the risk and decide if it is currently causing stress • Record the findings and decide on any action required to eliminate or reduce stress • Review the assessment over time

A. DEMANDS OF THE JOB	
• Work overload • Long hours • Proper rest and holidays • Inadequate staffing	• Prioritise tasks • Look at job design and working practices • Check leave is being properly taken. • Is work being taken home? Is there constant communication during off-duty time by email, text and phone? • Cut out unnecessary work and communications • Review workloads and staffing, and enable individuals to plan their work
• Inappropriately qualified for the job • Too little training for the job • Over promotion • Skills not recognised – promotion prospects not fulfilled	• Make sure individuals are matched to jobs – people can be over and under qualified • Analyse skills alongside the task • Provide training for those who need more, e.g. when introducing new technology • Review and consider selection, skill criteria, job summaries, training and supervision • Career planning discussion, training needs evaluation • Monitor workplace policies in practice: discrimination
• Boring or repetitive work	• Job enrichment/job rotation/role review • Assess workstation and work practice for possible solutions • Consider changing the way jobs are done by moving people between jobs, giving individuals more responsibility, increasing the scope of the job, increasing the variety of tasks, or giving a group of workers greater responsibility for effective performance of the group

• Inadequate resources for task	Analyse requirements for any project/task: • equipment/tools • staffing • priorities • deadlines
• Employees experiencing excessive workloads • Employees working under excessive pressure	• Review workload and demands regularly and as an integral part of the appraisal and performance management process • Support staff in planning their work. Try to establish what aspects of their job they find challenging. Redistribute work or set different work priorities if they are not coping • Check that holiday leave is being taken and staff needs are being accommodated • Check management skills and assess training needs
B. CONTROL OF WORK ENVIRONMENT	
• Not being able to balance the demands of work and life outside work	• Encourage a healthy work–life balance • Ensure staff take all their allocated holiday allowance and distribute it fairly across the year • Develop a communications protocol that ensures people have rest time completely free of all work-related messages. Over-anxious people often need to be in constant contact. Over-controlling management tends not to respect off-duty time
• Rigid work patterns • Fixed deadlines occurring in different parts of the year • Lack of control over work	• Try to provide some scope for varying working conditions and flexible work schedules (e.g. flexible working hours, working from home) • Consult with people to allow them to influence the way their jobs are done, what the real deadlines are and what the priorities are
• Conflicting work demands	• Set realistic deadlines for tasks • Take into account that individuals are different, and try to allocate work so that everyone is working in the way that helps them work best, takes account of their home obligations and makes best use of their skills • Be clear about tasks required
The physical working environment: • poor temperature control • noise • lack of facilities for rest/breaks • poor lighting • poor ventilation • badly placed or designed workstations	• Make sure workplace hazards are properly controlled • Undertake risk assessments of workspace and significant tasks

The psychological working environment: • threat of aggression or violence • verbal abuse • poor management practices	• Assess risks, implement controls including investigation of complaints and appropriate training • Monitor absence levels and trends. Compare with other departments, other businesses. • Look at the individual and any risk factors that apply to this particular person.

C. SUPPORT

• Return to work system • Sickness and absence management	• Policies and systems in place, monitored and consistently applied • Measure trends and changes • Investigate variations • Check management skills and assess training needs
• Inductions	• New staff properly inducted, existing staff transferring or promoted or returning to work after long absence also to be inducted • Special attention for young people as required • Mentoring roles • OH/HR support • DDA adjustments in place, reviewed and checked
• Post disciplinary, grievance or suspension	• Support staff as appropriate and in line with ACAS good practice

D. WORKPLACE RELATIONSHIPS

• Poor relationships with others • Staff complaints or rising absence trends	• Investigate causal factors • Provide training in interpersonal skills, non-discriminatory rules and workplace conduct standards • Discuss the problem openly with individuals • Follow complaint procedures • Check management skills and assess training needs
• Bullying or confrontational communication styles	• Encourage constructive and positive communications between staff • Managers should discuss and address bullying and/or confrontational communication styles with members of staff who display these behaviours • Consider training and policy guidance
• Bullying, racial or sexual harassment	• Set up effective systems to prevent bullying and harassment. Ensure staff are aware of the company's Dignity at Work Policy, which covers equal opportunities, stress problems, harassment, etc., and that they know how to get support or make a complaint • Practise by example and make it clear what behaviours are not acceptable • Provide details of any empirical evidence: absence trends, complaints, etc.

• Lack of support or fear culture within from management and co-workers.	• Support and encourage staff, protect them from reprisals • Consider introducing a mentoring and counselling scheme • Investigate and take action as appropriate as soon as possible

E. ROLE WITHIN ORGANISATION

• Clear lines of accountability and responsibility	• Ensure good communication systems exist and are in place from top to bottom • Set management standards to ensure best practice in: clarity of job function, responsibility for staff management and welfare • Make it clear to staff that management will try to ensure that their problems will be handled sensitively and at the appropriate level of management
• Lack of communication and consultation	• Communicate clear business objectives • Aim for good communication and close employee involvement, particularly during periods of change or high pressure
• A culture of blame when things go wrong, denial of potential problems • Failure to recognise success	• Be honest, set a good example, and listen to and respect others • Acknowledge and reward successes
• A culture that considers stress a sign of weakness	• Approachable management which wants to know about problems and will try to help to resolve them
• An expectation that people will regularly work excessively long hours or take work home with them	• Avoid working excessively long hours • Lead by example • Check management skills and assess training needs • Schedule work in a way that allows recovery time after unavoidable busy periods

F. MANAGEMENT OF CHANGE

• Fears about job security • Poor communication – uncertainty about what is happening • Not enough time allowed to implement change • Inexperience/fear of new technology • Lack of skills for new tasks • Not enough resource allocated for change process	• Provide effective support for staff throughout the process • Consult with staff likely to be involved in a change of management programme – fear and uncertainty can lead to increased anxiety, unfounded gossip, poor employment relationships and increased absence • Getting together as a team can help people to feel less isolated with their concerns • Ensure effective two-way communication throughout process – knowing exactly what is going to happen when can help people feel less anxious about a change • Consider training needs – do people have the tools and skills to effect change? • Consider environmental factors • Consider changes in teams or work environment – a small change, e.g. a different positioning of desks, can have a major impact on communication and work relationships to help people not to feel isolated

Appendix 11
Sample Protocol for Compliance with the Data Protection Act

To be reviewed and assessed against legal requirements, Code or Practice recommendations and organisational needs.

Principle 1
Data must be fairly and lawfully processed
	Applicable to recruitment
	
	• *Verification standards*
	   ◦ Give applicant the opportunity to rebut third party information.
	• *Pre-employment vetting*
	   ◦ Only vet where a job offer is to be made.
	   ◦ Ensure vetting is specific to the job and the individual and no more.
	   ◦ Ensure compliance with at least one of the sensitive data conditions where data is sought about family or close associates.
	• *Retention of recruitment records*
	   ◦ Obtain informed consent to retention of records for use for a potential further vacancy.
	
	Applicable to employment records
	
	• *Collection of information*
	   ◦ Inform new staff what information will be kept about them, where obtained, how used and circumstances where and to whom it may be disclosed.
	   ◦ Obtain informed consent to use of personal data.
	   ◦ Ensure that personal information is relevant and not excessive to the employment relationship.
	• *Maintaining records*
	   ◦ Ensure that personal information is relevant and not excessive to the employment relationship.
	• *Sickness records*
	   ◦ Only hold sickness records with explicit consent of the employee or if one of the other conditions for processing sensitive data is satisfied.
	   ◦ Explicit consent depends on each employee being told the extent of information that will be held in sickness records and how this will be used. Obtain evidence of consent.
	   ◦ Release of sickness records to managers should be limited to information reasonably required for management purposes.
	• *Occupational health schemes*
	   ◦ Obtain written consent to processing of data concerned with health. The employee must know the extent to which information given to a health professional directly or indirectly is made available to and used by others.

	Applicable to medical testing
	
	• *General standards*
	   ◦ Establish the specific business reason for testing.
	   ◦ Medical tests should be proportionate to the risk involved in failure to test whether by risk to others or to the individual concerned or if in relation to a health benefit such as sick pay.
	   ◦ Pre-employment medicals are justifiable to determine whether an employee is fit for the particular job or eligible to join a pension or insurance scheme.
	   ◦ Proportionate measures such as the use of a health questionnaire should be given first preference.
	   ◦ Only carry out tests on properly targeted employees unless blanket testing is justifiable.

Principle 2
Data must be processed for limited purposes and not in any manner incompatible with those purposes
	Applicable to recruitment
	
	• *Retention of recruitment records*
	   ◦ Vetting information should be kept securely until complete then destroyed, save for keeping a record that vetting has been carried out.
	
	Applicable to employment records
	
	• *Occupational health schemes*
	   ◦ Obtain written consent to processing of data concerned with health. The employee must know the extent to which information given to a health professional directly or indirectly is made available to and used by others.
	
	Applicable to medical testing
	
	• *General standards*
	   ◦ Establish the specific and genuine business reason for testing.

Principle 3
Data must be adequate, relevant and not excessive
	Applicable to recruitment
	
	• *Application form standards*
	   ◦ Require minimal personal information specific to the job in question.
	   ◦ State if information is to be taken from other sources.
	• *Pre-employment vetting*
	   ◦ Only carry out vetting if all other criteria for making a job offer have been satisfied.
	
	Applicable to employment records
	
	Tell new employees of their rights under the DPA 1998
	
	• *Collection of information*
	   ◦ Obtain informed consent to use of personal data and ensure that personal information is relevant and not excessive to the employment relationship.
	• *Occupational health schemes*
	   ◦ Obtain written consent to processing of data concerned with health. The employee must know the extent to which information given to a health professional directly or indirectly is made available to and used by others. Data must be processed in accordance with standards set out in the ethical guidelines of the Faculty of Occupational Medicine of the Royal College of Physicians.

	Applicable to medical testing
	
	• *General standards*
	  ○ Ensure testing is carried out as a necessary and proportionate matter to ensure there is no risk to health and safety of the individual or others or to secure a health benefit such as sick pay.
	  ○ Pre-employment medicals are justifiable to determine whether an employee is fit for the particular job or if eligible to join a pension or insurance scheme.
	  ○ Only carry out tests on properly targeted employees unless blanket testing is justifiable.
	  ○ Drug and alcohol testing should be part of a voluntary programme for detection of abuse.
	  ○ Substance testing should be by properly qualified persons.

Principle 4
Data must be accurate
	Applicable to recruitment
	
	• *Verification standards*
	  ○ Give applicant the opportunity to rebut third party information.
	• *Vetting*
	  ○ Ensure vetting is specific to the job and the individual and no more.
	  ○ Attempt to ensure accuracy where there is justification for obtaining information about the applicant's family or close associates as it will be difficult for them to rebut.
	
	Applicable to employment records
	
	• *Maintaining records*
	  ○ Ensure information in employee records is accurate and up to date. Good practice: provide every employee with a copy of his/her basic record annually and ask for identification of inaccuracies and what amendments are needed.
	  ○ Incorporate accuracy, consistency and validity checks.
	  ○ Require emergency contact not 'next of kin'.
	
	Applicable to medical testing
	
	• *General standards*
	  ○ Testing for drugs and alcohol should be by properly qualified persons. (*The Commission refers to tests of 'the highest technical quality' and to interpretation of results by a medically qualified person competent in the field of drug testing.*)

Principle 5
Data must not be kept for longer than necessary
	Applicable to recruitment
	
	• *Retention of recruitment records*
	  ○ Establish and adhere to retention periods for recruitment records where they need to be kept for business purposes. Suggested retention periods:
	    — 4 months from the date of confirmation of an unsuccessful application
	    — 4 months from the date of confirmation that another candidate was appointed to a short-listed position
	  ○ Vetting information should be kept securely until complete then destroyed, save for keeping a record that vetting has been carried out.

Principle 6
Data must be processed in accordance with the rights of the individual
	Applicable to recruitment
	Applicable to access and disclosure
	
	• *Subject access*
	   ○ Ensure that information is available within 40 days of the request being made and on receipt of the current £10 fee.
	   ○ Ensure that information is only released to the actual data subject.
	   ○ Provide information on file with reasons for why it is kept and explanation of any otherwise unintelligible terms.
	   ○ Ensure information is not provided that identifies other persons unless the third party consents to its release.
	• *References*
	   ○ Ensure identity of third party is not revealed.
	   ○ If third party information is integral to the reference, special procedures are set out in the Code Appendix allowing for consent by the third party or the overriding interest of the data subject.

Principle 7
Data must be kept securely
	Applicable to recruitment
	
	• *Application form standards*
	   ○ Provide secure method of transmission for on-line applications.
	   ○ State for whom data is being provided and how it will be used.
	
	Applicable to retention of records generally
	
	• *Standards of keeping sickness records*
	   ○ Release of sickness records to managers should be limited to information reasonably required for management purposes.
	• *Standards of security*
	   ○ Apply proper security standards as identified in BS7799 to protect from risk of accidental or unauthorised intervention leading to loss or destruction of or damage to employment records.
	   ○ Use system and password controls for information to be released to defined persons on a 'need to know basis'.
	   ○ Maintain a log and audit trail of all access to the records.
	   ○ Ensure reliability of staff having access to records.
	   ○ Unauthorised or otherwise improper access to records is a serious disciplinary offence and may also constitute a criminal offence.
	   ○ Take stringent precautions when transmitting data by e-mail or fax to ensure security encryption and receipt by the individual addressee.
	• *Occupational health schemes*
	   COMPLIANCE IS REQUIRED WITH THE STANDARDS SET OUT BY THE FACULTY OF OCCUPATIONAL MEDICINE
	   ○ Obtain written consent to processing of data concerned with health. The employee must know the extent to which information given to a health professional directly or indirectly is made available to and used by others.
	   ○ Security measures to be appropriate to the nature of sensitive data processed in connection with an occupational health scheme. Information should not be released even to occupational health professionals unless on a 'need to know' basis.

	Applicable to access to records
	
	• *Disclosure of references*
	   ○ Confidential references should not be given without the express consent of the subject to disclosure of the reference.
	• *Disclosure requests*
	   ○ Clear policies should be established and adhered to so as to ensure disclosure is only made to the proper subject who is entitled to access. Security measures include only accepting written requests and informing the Commissioner where it is suspected that an attempt is being made to obtain information by deception: **remember that there is no legal requirement to disclose even where a failure to do so would prejudice crime and taxation**.
	   ○ Disclosure should be by staff trained in data protection procedures.
	   ○ Records should be kept of non-routine disclosures.
	   ○ Disclosure records should be checked and procedures updated regularly.
	
	Remind staff regularly that disclosure to the wrong person is a criminal offence. It should be a disciplinary offence as well. Errors or deliberate releases of information should be reported to the Commissioner

Principle 8 Data must not be transferred to countries that do not have adequate protection.	**Exercise particular caution with any information transfers outside the European Economic Area and seek permission from employees in these circumstances.**

Glossary

Accountability To be answerable for the results of an assigned action. Accountability is associated with delegated authority and is distinct from responsibility. An employer can assign responsibility but cannot give away his/her accountability; the employer is ultimately accountable.

Clinical audit A quality improvement process that seeks to improve patient/client care and outcomes through systematic review of care against explicit criteria and the implementation of change.

Clinical governance A systematic approach to maintaining and improving the quality of patient/client care. It is intended to embody three key attributes: recognisably high standards of care, transparent responsibility and accountability for those standards, and a constant dynamic of improvement.

Curriculum vitae Sometimes abbreviated to CV, this is a document containing a summary or listing of professional education and qualifications, relevant job skills and experience.

Disability A physical or mental impairment that has a substantial and long-term adverse effect on one's ability to carry out normal day-to-day activities.

Discrimination To discriminate is to make a distinction. There are several meanings of the word, including statistical discrimination. The most common colloquial sense of the word is invidious discrimination, such as irrational social, racial, religious, sexual, ethnic and age-related discrimination of people.

Ergonomics Ergonomics (from Greek *ergon* work and *nomoi* natural laws) is the study of optimising the interface between human beings and the designed objects and environments with which they interact. It includes the study of workplace design and the physical and psychological impact it has on workers. Ergonomics is about the fit between people and their work activities, equipment, work systems and environment to ensure that workplaces are safe, comfortable and efficient.

Hazard Anything that can cause harm is a hazard, e.g. chemicals, electricity, using machinery.

Health assessment A one-to-one interaction between a client who is an employee or prospective employee, and an occupational health professional, usually a doctor or nurse, for the purposes of assessing the physical or mental status of the client.

Health screening A process by which undiagnosed diseases or defects are identified by tests.

Health surveillance The putting in place of systematic, regular and appropriate procedures to detect early signs of work-related ill health among employees exposed to certain health risks, and acting on the results.

Health record Any record that consists of information relating to the physical or mental health or condition of an individual, and has been made by or on behalf of a health professional in connection with the care of that individual. Health records cover the full range of media by which information can

	be held on an individual including, for example, scans, X-rays, printout results, computer records and handwritten notes.
Human resources	The department and support systems responsible for personnel sourcing and hiring, applicant tracking, skills development and tracking, benefits administration and compliance with associated government regulations.
Intranet	An interconnected network within one organisation that uses Web technologies for the sharing of information internally, not worldwide. Such information might include organisation policies and procedures, announcements, or information about new products.
Occupational hygiene	The discipline of anticipating, recognising, evaluating and controlling health hazards in the working environment with the objective of protecting worker health and well-being and safeguarding the community at large.
Rehabilitation	The process of helping a person to achieve the highest level of function, independence and quality of life possible.
Risk	The chance, high or low, that somebody will be harmed by a hazard.
Risk assessment	A careful examination of what could harm people in a given area or with a given task. The overall process is one of risk analysis and risk evaluation, and it is one step in the risk management process.
Vocational rehabilitation	An entitlement of a sick or injured employee to receive prompt rehabilitation and/or retraining, adjustments or job placement, as may be reasonably necessary to restore him or her to useful employment.

Index